JIM KARAS

THE ULTIMATE DIET REVOLUTION

Your Metabolism Makeover

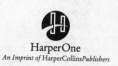

HarperOne
An Imprint of HarperCollinsPublishers

To Olivia and Evan

HarperOne

HarperCollins books may be purchased for educational, business, or sales promotional use. For information please e-mail the Special Markets Department at SPsales@harpercollins.com.

HarperCollins website: http://www.harpercollins.com

FIRST HARPERCOLLINS PAPERBACK EDITION PUBLISHED IN 2016

ISBN: 978-0-06-232158-9

Library of Congress Cataloging-in-Publication Data
Karas, Jim.
    The ultimate diet revolution : your metabolism makeover / Jim Karas.
      pages cm
    ISBN 978-0-06-232156-5 (hardcover)
    1. Reducing diets.   2. Metabolism—Regulation.   3. Physical fitness.   I. Title.
    RM222.2K3376   2015
    613.2'5—dc23
                                                          2015001631

16 17 18 19 20   RRD(H)   10 9 8 7 6 5 4 3 2 1

Contents

Introduction

You may have heard this staggering statistic. If one hundred people successfully lose weight, what percentage will have kept all the weight off after five years? Drumroll please. Five!!! Yep, the success rate is an incredibly *low* 5 percent, and that's the weight-loss world's "dirty little secret."

I myself have been part of this disheartening statistic. I spent the first twenty-one years of my life overweight, and sometimes *really* overweight. I can't tell you how many times I lost the weight, only to gain it back, and then some. But it was my fault, because each time I was telling—no, *demanding*—that my body gain the weight back. I would starve myself and then perform cardio, two behaviors that can ruin your metabolism. I was doing what I thought I should, but it was the exact opposite of what I actually should have been doing. In our nation, where obesity is on the rise, this is an all too common mistake that leads to our inability to keep the weight off.

Reading a statistic like this on weight-loss failure, you must be thinking, "Why even try? Donut, please!"

I'll tell you why you should—better yet, *must*—try. Because being at your optimal weight, even losing *any* weight, is essential to your health. I have been in the weight-loss business for over twenty years with an 80 percent success rate in helping clients not only lose weight but *keep the weight off.* My clients include movie and television stars you see all the time. Yep, I have the "secret" to successful, permanent weight loss, and it all revolves around one word: REVVED.

Let's start with the title of this book, *The Ultimate Diet REVolution*. Aristotle described a revolution as "a complete change from or modification of an existing constitution, . . . one that is such a motivating change in ideology that the masses follow."

Consider that, according to the Centers for Disease Control and Prevention, as of 2010:

- Of adults age twenty and over, 69.2 percent are considered overweight, which is defined as having a body mass index over 25 (only Mexico beats us with an overweight figure of 69.5 percent).

- Of that 69.2 percent who are overweight, 35.9 percent are obese, defined as having a body mass index of over 30.[1]

Sixty-nine percent clearly constitutes "the masses," and since the last time this number was determined was in 2010, I would say that it is even higher now and more people are part of this statistic. We are going the wrong way and continue to grow in size (no pun intended) every year. There is a 95 percent NON-success rate when it comes to weight loss. Don't you agree that it's time to *REV*olt?

REVVED is about *optimizing metabolism*. Every bit of research-backed advice I give you in the pages of this book has one simple, specific goal—*a* REVVED-*up metabolism*—and with that stoked metabolism comes the power to change your body and achieve permanent weight loss. I'm sure that many of you have tried and failed. I'm sure that some of you currently think that you can never achieve your ideal body. Metabolism is the key that unlocks all that you need in order to experience incredible weight-loss success. You already have the power *within* you.

Metabolism is the chemical change in living cells that creates the energy necessary for being physically active—and for simply staying alive. Our *REVVED* goal is to stoke those "chemical processes" up and get them running at full speed. Think of yourself as a powerful convertible sports car. You want your motor racing as you "run out" each gear and speed along the highway, the top down and your hair whipping in the wind. I want your metabolism *REVVED* just like that sexy car. And that can happen at *any* age and at *any* time. It's not too late—you're in charge of your body, your metabolism, and your future.

You see, it isn't inevitable for your metabolism to become sluggish or devolve into what many people term a *slow* metabolism. How many times have I heard "Oh, I just have a slow metabolism. It runs in my family." But that's not true. What your metabolism is doing is listening and responding to your instructions, which are dictated by your beliefs and behaviors. The truth is that YOU are in control of your metabolism. Your metabolism doesn't control you.

A note about belief in a bad, or slow, metabolism because of genes: Some people eat often, they eat the wrong foods, and their subsequent inability to take the weight off reinforces their belief that their metabolism is stacked against them. It's a terribly destructive cycle that has to be broken—and breaking it is one of my goals with this book. I will go into the genetic component of a *REVVED* metabolism in chapter 2.

I'm going to teach you a new belief system about your body and your weight. Your new belief will then result in success-driven behaviors. Did you notice that I said "behaviors"? Not just one behavior, but many—a completely new way of approaching your body. Presto: weight loss, and this time—and this is a huge point—*all* the weight you lose is fat loss, not muscle loss. You will learn how to control what occurs within your mind, which leads to changes in your body. You do so by making new *REVVED* choices.

Here's an example. Do you believe that it's okay to skip breakfast? If so, then that belief and subsequent behavior (having just coffee or, worse, a glass of juice) increases your odds of becoming overweight or obese by 450 percent.[2]

Why? Skipping breakfast disrupts your metabolism and actually reduces it by between 5 and 10 percent. This slowing down happens because the human body is very, very smart. When you skip breakfast, the body wonders, "Why aren't I being fed? There must not be a readily available source of food around. This could go on for some time, so I better slow my metabolism down so I can stay alive on fewer calories."

How does the body efficiently go about slowing itself down? It draws from its most metabolically active tissue: muscle. You instantly start to lose your *REVVED* efficient metabolism. Start believing that eating breakfast is essential, then change your behavior (make sure to eat breakfast each and every day, and make it a BIG meal), and that devastating metabolic reduction starts to *REV*erse. And the exciting part is that you start to get *REVVED* back immediately.

And those of you who simply say "I'm not hungry in the morning," do you know why you aren't hungry? It's for one of two reasons:

1. Your smart brain got tired of asking for food in the morning. After not getting it for days, weeks, months, or maybe even years, the brain

said, "Enough. Don't ask, 'cause you're not gonna get it." Your body listened to your instructions.

2. You gorged the night before and your body is still dealing with the onslaught of a huge dinner, then dessert, then snacking. Sound familiar?

It's not only your metabolism that you are killing by skipping breakfast. You actually up the odds of killing yourself. Skipping breakfast may lead to obesity, high blood pressure, high cholesterol, and diabetes. In fact, men who skipped breakfast regularly increased the odds of dying from a heart attack or stroke by 27 percent.[3]

Women don't escape breakfast-skipping consequences either, as a very large study in the *American Journal of Clinical Nutrition* showed. Women who skipped just one breakfast a week increased their risk of developing type 2 diabetes by 20 percent.[4]

I'm going to ask you to change your belief. I'm going to ask you to acknowledge that eating breakfast is essential to having an efficient and fully energized metabolism. And I'm going to ask you to put that belief into action by planning to eat within the same 30-minute window every single day, Monday through Sunday. I will give you more details and the research behind this part of my plan, but just know that your body *loves* routine and responds by trusting you to take good care of it. It likes to know when it's going to get up, when it's going to eat, when it's going to rest, and so on. Compelling research shows big results from a structured approach. Make a habit of eating at the same time, and your body won't have to override your actions. Working *with* your body rather than against it really helps speed up the weight-loss process and, more important, keeps the weight off.

Think of how much a newborn likes routine and a schedule. Ideally, you put the baby down to sleep at the same time each night. When the baby wakes up, he or she is ready to eat and eats as much as is needed. You burp the baby, and then it's a little playtime, a good poop, and soon nap time. It's like clockwork: sleep, eat, burp, play, poop, sleep. I was amazed at how happy, nonfussy, and smiley my own children, Olivia and Evan, were when on their schedule. I'm sure you have experienced the same with your own children or others you have spent time around. Now, when my kids weren't on their schedule—well, have you seen Chucky in *Child's Play*?

I love smart, quick results, but they need to last forever. Who wants to lose 15 pounds, only to gain 20 back? Is that you? Haven't we all done that in the past? Now, with this book, you finally have all the data you need to make lasting changes. While you're reading, I hope you will experience that "aha" moment when it all makes sense. You will nod your head and think, "Why didn't I realize this before?" It's okay. You don't have to figure it out for yourself. That's my job. That's why people hire my firm, Jim Karas Personal Training, in Chicago and New York in addition to utilizing my Skype training all over the world. It's really not complicated, because

- my method gets results;

- results bring attention;

- attention translates to referrals; and

- referrals flow from both clients and their physicians, who keep asking me, "What is it that you do that's so effective? All my patients who go to you are in better shape than they were in their twenties."

I have spent over twenty years in the trenches, working with clients multiple times a week for multiple years and teaching my staff new techniques, new eating plans, new stress-relief behaviors, and all that clients need to achieve true success. I also depend on research—I cite a lot of it in this book. But if I can't get clients to "buy into" my plan and truly change their beliefs and behaviors, all the research in the world is not going to motivate them to take action. I have to get into the client's head. I have to get into *your* head. My goal is to make you a believer in my established, success-driven plan for permanent weight and fat loss.

This is my sixth book. Four out of my past five books were *New York Times* bestsellers, and I'm extremely proud to have helped readers reach their goals while proving some of the most popular weight-loss myths to be untrue. I have helped readers come up with concrete plans, get their energy back, overcome excuses once and for all, and create real and lasting change in their lives. In many ways, this book is a culmination and continuation of all five of my prior books, but it offers so much more. As I said earlier, in the past few years, my firm has grown considerably. It has done so because of the 80 percent success rate I previously alluded to. We call these results "transformations." We actually rate our staff of personal fitness trainers by how many transformations they accomplish each quarter. It's a part of our review process. That's the value we put on results, and we're getting more of them than ever before with *REVVED* solutions.

I've pounded home the whole concept of *REVVED* beliefs and behaviors as the foundation of these transformations. My clients keep the weight off *and* significantly change their body's composition. It therefore became so

I want to address the National Weight Control Registry's definition of weight-loss success. The Registry is a population of more than four thousand individuals who are over eighteen and have lost approximately 30 pounds and kept it off for at least a year. They disagree with my suggested very low success rate of 5 percent and believe it's truly closer to 20 percent. This makes more sense when you realize that they "define" success as losing 10 percent of your body weight (or more) and keeping it off for a year. But if you are a 300-pound man and manage to lose 10 percent of your body weight, or the 30 pounds mentioned above, you still weigh 270 pounds. Although every pound lost is a victory for your health, helping to reduce the risk of diabetes, heart disease, and cancer, I am concerned that by setting only a modest goal, you may be setting the bar too low.

Plus, the Registry acknowledges that many of the people who have lost 10 percent of their weight may still be, by definition, obese. I think that's the reality. We aren't talking about a lot of size-8 women or men with 32-inch waists. I by no means am telling you that you have to have a body that could be on the cover of a health or sports magazine. I'm saying let's get out (and stay out) of the overweight and obese categories. Let's also not stop with only a 10 percent reduction in body weight if your health and fitness level truly calls for more. Let's make our goal a smart, lean one. And fix our sights on your best weight and lean-muscle mass.

The Registry also does not take into consideration body composition. As you will soon learn, when the vast majority of people lose weight, at least half of it is muscle, maybe more. So those who have done nothing but decimate their muscle and metabolism are called "success" stories. Plus, if people strength-train, which is a core component of *REVVED* behavior, they keep their muscle or increase it, which is our goal and which may not always mean weight loss, but will mean fat loss.

The other major problem with the Registry is that it's self-reported. Come on—how many of us tell the absolute truth about our weight? I know I didn't when I was overweight. Self-reported studies truly cannot be held up as fact. There is just too much temptation to fudge the truth. Who wants to report that they gained the weight back? Not many people.[5]

abundantly clear to me that this was the next logical book for me to write, as I truly do want to expand the *REV*olution that I've started in Chicago and New York, throughout the country, and beyond.

When you start this plan, you will immediately see and feel a real difference in your body. It's exciting and motivating.

What will you see? A leaner, lighter, tighter you, and—maybe for the first time ever—you will see your body's composition changing. How thrilling! And you're never going back to how you used to be. Why? Because you're performing an exercise program that completely reshapes your body. Just think of what it would look like to have a tighter physique; lean, toned arms and legs; great posture; and flat, hard abs, regardless of your age, regardless of your body type. What would it be like to throw open your closet and realize that your "slim" clothes fit? Or better yet, that you have to buy new clothes that show off your new body. You don't have the angst of figuring out what *might* fit, what suit jacket or pants *might* button or skirt *might* zip up. Trust me—after having tons of clothes in the past that correlated to my ever changing weight, it's just great living lean in each and every way.

What will you feel? Energized, happy, and finally convinced that this is *the* plan you can stick with for life. You will leave your old body behind and never look back.

I want it all for you. And I will help you get there.

I'm a big fan of crime-scene shows. My favorite part is when one of the investigators figures out that "aha" piece of evidence that was previously overlooked or misunderstood. That's what solves the case. You may be wondering, "Why do I struggle at weight loss, and then the moment I manage to shed a few pounds, they all come right back and then some?" The *REVVED* plan will help you find that "aha" moment where you see what the evidence is telling you and everything becomes clear.

Get ready for your *REV*olution. Prepare yourself for a new belief system that will be supported by the evidence you are about to uncover.

In the beginning of this book, I'm going to explain the secrets of weight loss, the whole concept of a *REVVED* body, and how certain beliefs and behaviors dictate the direction of your weight and metabolism.

Next, you'll discover why most diets, and especially cleanses, destroy metabolism and how you can restore yours.

Then I will present my eating rules and a detailed, 28-day eating plan. It's a classic plan covering all food groups, including meat and dairy, but I have also provided vegetarian and gluten-free options, as so many people have asked me for them.

After that will come the exercise rules and the 32-minute exercise routine that can be performed in your home, office, exercise facility, or anywhere you can find a small space. Why 32 minutes? Well, you'll have to wait to find out. This exercise routine will use a new product I have developed. It's inexpensive, simple to use, and astonishingly effective.

Finally, I will outline the residual benefits of this plan, which include a more energized, smarter, trimmer, and younger you.

So, fasten your seat belt, hit the gas, and get ready to conquer weight loss once and for all.

Simply put—get ready to be *REVVED*.

REVVED by the Numbers

Metabolism. It's a word we often use when we talk about losing weight, but what is it really? Let's go back to the definition of metabolism I gave in the introduction: *"the chemical change in living cells that creates the energy necessary for being physically active."*

Now let's build on that. *Metabolism* is also defined as

> The sum total of the chemical processes that occur in living organisms, resulting in growth, production of energy, elimination of waste material, etc.[1]

Taking this one step further, every person possesses a *basal metabolic rate*, which is defined as

> The amount of energy required by an individual in the resting state, for such functions as breathing and circulation of the blood.[2]

Think of it this way. Even when your car is in park and idling, it is still burning gas. The same applies to your body. Even when you are sleeping, your body continues to require a certain number of calories to keep it functioning

---

REVVED Fiction   "You don't have to count calories to lose weight." Wrong! I like what the *Journal of the American Dietetic Association* says about that claim: "Whenever you see a diet book or article that says you don't have to count calories—run!"

REVVED Fact   A calorie is a unit of energy. The calories you take in provide the "fuel" your body uses to "run." If you are over your desirable weight, then you have simply "overfueled," and your body has stored those extra calories as fat. It takes 3,500 calories to equal 1 pound of fat.

---

properly and enable all of the nightly repair work that the body requires. It is calories that keep you alive and provide the energy necessary for your most basic bodily functions.

Even though the *REVVED* Eating Plan is calorie-based, *you* don't have to worry about counting calories; I've already done all that work for you.

Calculating Your Basal Metabolic Rate (BMR)

You may be wondering, "How do I find out what my basal metabolic rate is—that is, the number of calories I need if I rest all day and do no activity at all?" It's hard to obtain the precise number, but you can get an approximate one by using the Harris-Benedict Equation, which is:

Women: BMR = 655 + (4.35 × **weight in pounds**) + (4.7 × **height in inches**) − (4.7 × **age in years**)

Men: BMR = 66 + (6.23 × **weight in pounds**) + (12.7 × **height in inches**) − (6.8 × **age in years**)

For example, I'm 175 pounds, six feet tall, and fifty-three years old, so when I fill in my equation it looks like this:

66 + (6.23 × 175) + (12.7 × 72) − (6.8 × 53) or

66 + 1,090.25 + 914.4 − 360.4 = 1,710.25

That's how many calories my body would burn on a daily basis if I just lay down and did nothing.

Now let's calculate your basal metabolic rate.

WOMEN

Your weight in pounds:	_____
× 4.35	
Total:	_____
Your height in inches:	_____
× 4.7	
Total:	_____
Your age in years:	_____
× 4.7	
Total:	_____

Add totals from 1, 2, and 3: _____

+ 655

Total: _____ = your BMR

MEN

Your weight in pounds: _____

× 6.23

Total: _____

Your height in inches: _____

× 12.7

Total: _____

Your age in years: _____

× 6.8

Total: _____

Add totals from 1, 2, and 3: _____

+ 66

Total: _____ = your BMR

Calculating Your Active Metabolic Rate (AMR)

Now you want to calculate what is termed your *active metabolic rate* (AMR). This will give you the number of calories needed for your basal metabolic functions *and* your daily movement and exercise.

Calculate your active metabolic rate by starting with your basal metabolic rate and adjusting it with one of these multipliers by estimating your current level of activity. If you are:

Sedentary
(little or no exercise)

BMR × 1.2 = AMR

Lightly Active
(light exercise/work 1 to 3 days per week)

BMR × 1.375 = AMR

Moderately Active
(moderate exercise/work 3 to 5 days per week)

BMR × 1.55 = AMR

Very Active
(hard exercise/work 6 to 7 days per week)

BMR × 1.725 = AMR

Extra Active   BMR × 1.9 = AMR
(*very* hard exercise/work 6 to 7 days per week)

A few points: I bet the "Lightly Active" multiplier probably pertains to you. If your activity is a short walk to work or your transportation to work, or if you perform some exercise a couple of times a week and do the usual housework, shopping, errand running, and so forth, then this is you.

Personally, I use the "Moderately Active" multiplier, as I work out about 3 hours a week (I bet you thought it would be more—I will explain why it isn't in chapter 7) and walk everywhere. Still, I don't think it's right for me to use the "Very Active" multiplier. If you don't exercise but live in a classic walking city like New York, Chicago, London, or Paris, and you actually *walk* to things, then I'm fine with your saying that you are moderately active even without any structured exercise.

My definition of a person who may use the "Very Active" multiplier would be your classic Beverly Hills housewife. She takes yoga virtually every morning, then plays tennis with her pro in the afternoon three times a week. On the other afternoons, she sees her trainer for an hour of strength training or Pilates. She is exercising in one form or another for 1 to 2 hours a day almost every day. Just for the record, I don't think this is a smart strategy at all (it's actually a stress-inducing, injury-provoking, aging one), and I will tell you why later in the book.

The "Extra Active" multiplier only applies if you are Lance Armstrong in his heyday, cycling like a crazy man on a daily basis; Michael Phelps swimming "turbo" laps all morning; or one of the Williams sisters training for the finals at Wimbledon. It's rare that nonserious athletes can use that number, so try to avoid it.

And finally, please don't use your *aspirational* activity level. Use the multiplier that truly represents how much you *presently* move and exercise. Sure, in the future, that will probably change, but for now, let's be honest.

As an example, my active metabolic rate is:

1,710.25 (BMR) × 1.55 (Activity Multiplier) = 2,651 (yes, I rounded up a few tenths of a percent)

That means that I need 2,651 calories a day to maintain my weight at my current level of activity.

Now let's calculate your AMR.

Your BMR is _____

Your Activity Multiplier is _____

Your BMR multiplied by
your Activity Multiplier is _____ = your AMR

Keep your AMR in mind when we talk about what you need to eat to lose weight in chapter 4; we will revisit this number.

You can have your basal metabolic rate tested on a $50,000 piece of equipment called the Bod Pod. This "pod" is a giant egg that you sit in to determine your body-fat percentage and basal metabolic rate. The technology used is called air-displacement plethysmography. It's fast, and it has been found to be quite accurate. You may find a Bod Pod at a university or hospital in your area. Try a Google search. A single test usually runs between $25 and $100.[3]

For the average, sedentary American, the basal metabolic rate makes up approximately 60 percent of the active metabolic rate. Digestion accounts for the next 10 percent and relates to the "thermic effect" of food. This thermic effect gauges how much energy it takes to break down and digest the food you consume. Certain foods (like protein) possess a much higher thermic effect, and a high thermic effect plays right into our *REVVED* strategy. (This will be detailed in chapter 4.) The remaining 30 percent of AMR in this sedentary example is from nonexercise activity thermogenesis, or NEAT.

Please note this is for sedentary people and not for those who do structured exercise, especially the style of exercise I will encourage you to perform.

REVVED Fiction "Hormones do not play a role in how your body processes calories taken in and calories expended." Yes, hormones do (more on that in chapter 4). Your hormones dictate how your body gains and loses weight as much as your activity level and what you eat do.

REVVED Fact Regardless of age, you have the ability to alter your metabolism in a positive (or negative) way.

I find that men and women respond similarly when I point out the fact that their current body weight is the function of every calorie they have ever consumed minus their calories out.

When I have a woman in her fifties at an initial consultation, the conversation generally goes something like this:

> "So, Mrs. Smith, why do you think you are at your present weight?"

> Mrs. Smith sits up, hands folded, legs crossed, leans into my desk, and says, "Well, Jim, you know I have children."

> "Oh, how wonderful. How old are they?"

> "Twenty-six and twenty-four."

Really? Twenty-four years ago you gave birth, and that's the reason for your present body weight? You must believe the "research" that says you have six months to get all the baby pounds off or they will literally "hang around" forever? Those baby pounds should have dropped off decades ago.

Now for the men:

> "So, Mr. Jones, why do you think you are at your present weight?"

> Mr. Jones, a sixty-four-year-old retired attorney, inhales, looks me straight in the eye, also leans in like Mrs. Smith, and proclaims with conviction, "You know, Jim, when I was in my early forties I had a really stressful, long case that included a lot of travel."

Really? Twenty years ago you had a stressful case, and now you're a good 45 pounds (I'm being kind; more like 65 pounds) overweight? I don't think so.

In both instances, the person believed there was a single reason why he or she was overweight. But the truth is that for long periods of time they behaved in such a way that kept the extra weight on. It was not pregnancy or one bad, stressful stretch of time. Our bodies are dynamic, constantly prepared to change whenever we give them the cues to change!

Enough about past behavior, which neither you nor I can do anything about. Instead, let's look at the present, which we can change.

Starting now.

Your present body weight is a function of the following equation:

Calories In (Food & Drink) − Calories Out (Activity & BMR) = Your Present Body Weight

You should interpret this equation to mean that, in the present, if you weigh approximately 150 pounds, then your calories in minus calories out results in a 150-pound body weight on the scale. If that is your desired weight, congratulations! If your true goal is to weigh 140 pounds, then it's a good thing that you have this book in your hands. If you *believe* you are dieting and the scale is not moving, well, honestly, your *behavior* is not getting the job done. You're not on a weight-loss plan or diet. It is great that you are making an effort, but it isn't an effective effort that will result in what you desire. You are really on "a maintenance."

The exception to this is those who are dramatically changing their body's composition via strength training. The scale may be saying " maintenance," but the fact that your body is shrinking, your abs are flattening, and your whole body is looking long and lean indicates that you are doing a wonderful job of burning body fat and replacing it with lean, calorie-burning muscle tissue. That means your calories-in-and-calories-out equation is changing too. In other words, your body is becoming more efficient and your calories are being used to feed your muscle rather than being stored as fat.

But, if you aren't strength-training and your weight keeps increasing, then you are on "a weight gain." To lose weight, you have to create a quality caloric deficit. Note the word "quality," as quality food is essential to the *REVVED* Eating Plan.

REVVED math works a little differently, as you will see in a moment. We are *REVO*lutionizing arithmetic (that's my secret), so we are actually going to redefine your "calories in" as we

- increase the number of quality calories in your diet; and

- decrease low-value calories, as they are causing a myriad of hormonal issues and preventing you from shedding fat.

And we are going to redefine your "calories out" as we

- eliminate the enormous amount of time you are wasting slaving away at cardiovascular exercise; and

- add interval-based strength training, as it increases your metabolism, melts fat for good, and provides a huge afterburn, so that your body will burn more calories 24 hours a day, 7 days a week, and continue to do so as long as you keep up your *REVVED* behaviors.

We are also going to manipulate your *REV*olutionary equation with hormonal balance, which will work for you instead of against you, as it did before you adopted *REVVED* behaviors.

When you start this plan, you will immediately create a caloric deficit by eating the right *REVVED* foods, so that the weight will quickly start to fall off and stay off. But this time, you will be hormonally balanced, creating an environment exclusively for fat loss, while preserving muscle and increasing your metabolism rather than letting it decrease. When you follow my eating and exercise plan and adopt all *REVVED* behaviors, you get *REVVED up* and your metabolism literally explodes (in a great way), so that you burn more calories 24 hours a day, 7 days a week, 365 days a year. The beauty of this strategy is that it doesn't stop *REV*ing until you tell it stop. As long as you follow this plan, you will optimize your *REVVED*-up body regardless of your age. That's right—age doesn't matter. *REVVED* behaviors trump age.

> You may know someone who says "I can eat whatever I want, because I have a good metabolism." I believe that can be true. I also believe people who eat whatever they want have a diet that consists mostly of what I call "clean" foods—lean protein, nuts, fruits, and vegetables—with a little bit of everything else, but not much. They also are consistent exercisers and are hormonally in balance. I'm sorry, but people who live "lean," with optimal *REVVED* bodies, don't live on what I call "crap cubed," which is the *c* trifecta: carbs, cardio, and confusion. ("Really, that deep-dish piece of pizza was 2,271 calories? I had no idea!") They live a far more *REVVED*-aware lifestyle.

Once again, I had it all wrong for so many years. I never gave metabolism a thought. I just focused on how aerobic exercise was going to get my weight off. My earliest memories were of what family members and friends referred to as my "cute" pot belly. Please, never, ever make a comment to a child or young person like that, as we know it's *not* cute. And that early pain and humiliation can lead to deadly eating disorders later in life.

I jumped rope in my basement. I did jumping jacks. (I'm sure that was *not* a pretty sight.) I ran in place, as I was too embarrassed to do it outside, and quite frankly in the late 1960s and early 1970s most people weren't doing that either. Then, in 1977, Jim Fixx's first book, *The Complete Book of Running*, was published. All of a sudden, the streets, the running tracks, and the treadmills were packed with those of us who thought, "Aha! Now I have the answer to losing weight and getting lean."

Aha, we had the answer—NOT!

What a disaster. I did it. I bought into that false belief that "cardio will make me lean," and I behaved as if it would actually work. It didn't. It didn't for most Americans. Again, with 69.2 percent of people overweight, and 35.9 percent of those obese, we are clearly failing. But the number of people performing cardio goes up every year.

Do Calories Burned During Exercise Matter?

I always looked at the "calories burned" window on any piece of cardio equipment I mounted. To be honest, I fixated on it. I was so proud when I stayed on the stair stepper or treadmill until I burned lots and lots of calories, upwards of 1,000. "Wow!" I thought. "Look at me." I was so proud of myself. But those numbers were and are a complete and utter lie. They're fiction, and here's research supporting my claim.

The University of California at San Francisco's Human Performance Center used a VO_2 analyzer, called New Leaf, to track calories burned during exercise. Part of this technology includes a facemask that resembles what Darth Vader wore in the *Star Wars* movies. Remember hearing his breathing? Same concept. That's how they measure the calorie burn. What the researchers found was a bit shocking (but not to me):

1. Calories burned on the treadmill were overestimated by 12 percent.

2. Calories burned on the stationary bike were overestimated by 7 percent.

3. Calories burned on the stair climber were overestimated by 12 percent.

4. Calories burned on the elliptical trainer were overestimated by— drumroll please—42 percent.[4]

For years I have called the elliptical trainer the "weapon of mass distraction." The reason is that the manufacturer of the first machine clearly *knew* that people fixated on the number of *supposed* calories expended. Therefore, it jacked up the display of number of calories burned. Wrong! A machine can never know, even when you plug in your height, weight, and age, how many calories you are burning. Only this very specific Darth Vader piece of technology can do that for you.

Now, since this research, I believe most newer machines have followed suit and increased the number of calories on the display to make them appear more efficient at achieving a fictitious calorie burn. The cardio rooms stay packed with a lot of struggling people on the machines, burning hours—not calories—clinging to both the guardrails *and* the belief that it will work.

It won't. It can't.

I want you to fixate on the calories you are going to burn through *REVVED* behaviors, not through some inaccurate machine. We aren't going to make that mistake. Instead, we are going to fixate on the number of calories you burn 24 hours a day, both during exercise and, even more important, *after* you are finished. That's when *REVVED* magic really begins.

I want you to embrace the term "*after*burn."

The Seven Secrets of REVVED

In my study of metabolism and development of the *REVVED* program, I have discovered seven basic components of *REV*ing it up that everyone should know before they get started.

REVVED Component Number 1: Muscle

The foundation of the *REVVED* program is a set of core beliefs and behaviors that optimize metabolism and your hormonal balance to facilitate weight and fat loss.

REVVED **Fiction**   "Muscle weight is different from fat weight." That's not true, but what is true is that 1 pound of muscle takes up less space than 1 pound of fat.

REVVED **Fact**   One pound of muscle burns 6 calories per day, and 1 pound of fat burns 2 calories per day.[1] Six calories for muscle versus 2 calories for fat doesn't seem like much of a difference. But trust me, it's a *huge* one with regard to metabolism, and that seemingly small difference adds up to a life of "living lean" rather than "living large."

We are going to augment your body's composition so that you not only maintain and increase muscle while eliminating fat but truly change the whole way your body is proportioned.

There are two basic types of fat, subcutaneous and visceral, and a third that might be called a fat condition:

1. **Subcutaneous fat is found directly under the skin.** This is the fat that you may pinch when thinking "I really need to lose some weight" (which is what I do when I'm up a few pounds and feel the "love handles"

on the sides of my abdominals), and it is the majority of fat that is measured using an old-fashioned body-fat-percentage method, such as calipers.

2. **Visceral fat is the fat that wraps around the internal organs.** It is believed that visceral fat is the far more dangerous of the two fats because of its proximity to the internal organs. It also is believed to play a greater role in a condition called insulin resistance, as visceral fat cells produce certain hormones, such as adiponectin, which is thought to influence the response of cells to insulin. (You will understand much more regarding the role of insulin and its effect on all types of body fat in subsequent chapters.) Visceral fat is also tricky. Some men and women who don't have visible fat but very large thighs or abdomens say to me, "Look at me. I'm all muscle," when in reality they are all fat. Instead of jiggling, it's solidly wrapped around their organs and muscles.

3. **The third type of fat, which I recognize and call a fat condition, is belly fat, and it's a combination of visceral and subcutaneous fat.** Across the board, physicians agree that belly fat is the most lethal to both your mind and body. A preponderance of belly fat has shown to accelerate dementia, so clearly it is not good for the mind. As for the body, insulin resistance, unhealthy blood lipids, and an increased risk of heart disease and stroke are some of the damaging conditions that arise as a result of this combination of fat in and around the belly.

The great news is that this *REVVED* strategy is a fat buster—all types of fat. It especially targets that dangerous belly fat. This comprehensive eating, exercise, and lifestyle plan is all about shedding fat forever.

REVVED Component Number 2: Genes

I have already mentioned the fact that the majority of overweight people I meet are convinced that their present weight is primarily attributable to their genes.

The *New York Times* reported on several research studies that examined the relationship between genes and body weight. One very provocative bit of research was done with three baby mice from the same parents. All three were fed the same number of calories, but one mouse grew to be twice the size of its siblings, and that additional size was all fat. In the large mouse, the researchers had deleted a gene known as MRAP2, which decreases the speed at which calories are burned. That decreased the "calories out" part of the equation. This gene is also called a "helper" gene, since it signals another gene known to control appetite. Once the helper gene was removed, appetite increased substantially, and the "calories in" part increased.

When the mice were young, the mouse with the deleted gene was controlled by the scientists so that it ate approximately 10 to 15 percent *fewer* calories than its siblings to stay at the same, lean weight. But once puberty hit, the appetite of the soon-to-be obese mouse became uncontrollable. That voracious appetite caused the doubling in size.[2]

But when it comes to humans, to date only one known morbidly obese child presented with the same deleted gene—only one. If you or someone you know also was or is a morbidly obese child, then genetic testing may make sense, but the chances that the obesity is caused by this missing gene are going to be infinitesimal.

In a second study, Dr. Claude Bouchard, a genetics researcher at the Pennington Biomedical Research Center in Baton Rouge, Louisiana, looked at twelve pairs of lean identical twins. They were kept in an enclosed facility, so that all exercise, nonexercise activity, and food were carefully monitored. He overfed them by 1,000 calories a day. The results showed that both twins in each set gained the same amount of weight, but some sets gained only 9½ pounds, while others gained as much as 29. That's a threefold difference.[3] Clearly there must have been some other condition affecting the outcome, such as:

A hormonal imbalance. If the hormones leptin, ghrelin, or insulin, to name a few, are not properly firing, this would affect weight gain or loss.

A larger proportion of lean muscle tissue. Twins possessing more lean, calorie-burning muscle will clearly have a higher metabolism and therefore gain less weight than those with less muscle.

The amount of sleep experienced each night, as that perpetuates the hormonal imbalance if less than seven to eight hours.

The percentage of brown fat to white fat. When stimulated, brown fat actually burns white fat. Brown fat is often called "a heat-generating type of fat that *burns* energy instead of storing it."[4] Some researchers place muscle and brown fat in the same category, because they provide similar functions when it comes to burning calories and white fat (which is your *REVVED* goal).

Brown fat is beginning to receive more and more attention these days. Endocrinologist Aaron Cypess, a professor at Harvard Medical School and research associate at the Joslin Diabetes Center in Boston, says: "Although leaner adults have more brown fat than heavier people, even their brown fat cells are greatly outnumbered by white fat cells. A 150-pound person might have 20 or 30 pounds of fat, but they are only going to have 2 or 3 ounces of brown fat. But that 2 ounces, if maximally stimulated, could burn off 300 to 500 calories a day—enough to lose up to a pound in a week."[5]

Sounds like "calories in" minus "calories out" might have to be challenged, since it is clearly not a matter of simple math.

A third study asked: Does exercise trump genetics? People inherit variations of the fat-mass or obesity-associated gene FTO, nicknamed by the researchers the "fatso" gene. When looking at more than 218,000 people with at least one copy of the FTO variation, researchers learned that for them the risk of becoming an obese adult increased by 30 percent. But people who had only one copy of the gene and exercised cut their risk of adult obesity to 22 percent, which represents a 27 percent reduction.

For those who possessed two or more copies of the FTO gene, the risk of becoming an obese adult increased to 70 percent. But once again, those who had two or more copies of the gene and exercised reduced the risk to 49 percent, a 30 percent reduction.

What was surprising to me was the form of exercise that these individuals performed to reduce their obesity risk. It was simple, nonintense movement, such as 30 minutes of walking the dog, riding a bike, or tending a garden. They performed these nonintense movements five days a week.[6]

Another study, reported in the *Archives of Internal Medicine* in 2008, explored a community of Amish people with the FTO gene variations. All they had to do to trump their genetics and stay lean was to perform their daily chores.[7]

What is my takeaway from these three studies? With regard to the first, as previously noted, only one young morbidly obese child has ever been found to have the deleted gene. I do believe, however, that there is an obesity gene or family of genes, like the FTO genes. I have known one family that clearly has a genetic curse working against many members. Now, some members clearly fall into the morbidly obese category (people who are more than 100 pounds overweight); they have given up even trying to make wise food choices or attempting to exercise. Other members of the family who started off heavier have successfully kept themselves almost lean, not even overweight. How did they prevail against their genetic programming? They balanced their hormones with a smart, "clean" eating plan, slept between 7 and 8 hours a night, minimized stress, and performed interval-based strength training with intensity. Funny—that's exactly what you are going to do on the *REVVED* plan.

In the twins study, if you dig into the research, all the twins supposedly started out lean and then were overfed 1,000 calories a day. First, flip the research and don't overfeed them. Would they all have stayed lean, since they started out lean? "Probably" is my answer, unless some of them just came off a significant weight loss. Weight loss changes the environment and brings hormonal imbalance into the equation, which would make it far more likely that they might gain some or all of that weight back.

> Past perfect or past imperfect? That's an important question to ask with regard to many of the components of this plan. If you haven't made the right food choices in the past, haven't slept well in years, have lived in a highly stressed state, or have never really exercised with intelligence or planning, then the odds are it may be a little harder for you to lose weight. But—and trust me on this—the moment you embrace each and every *REVVED* behavior, you *will* begin to lose weight.

With regard to the third study, as I've just made clear, exercise trumps the "bad genes" argument. Remember, most of the people in the study who "exercised" simply walked the dog, rode a bike, or did daily chores. That reduced the risk of obesity somewhat. When you hear more about the *REVVED* Exercise Plan, you will understand that I don't call those activities (walking the dog, riding a bike) exercise. I call them "active rest"—but more on that later.

Research conducted by Dr. Jonathan Ruiz shows that the "negative effects" of the FTO gene "disappeared" for *active* adolescents. Those adolescents actually resembled teens who did not carry the FTO gene.[8] Remember, it was nicknamed the "fatso" gene, but exercise appears to have renamed it the "fat—NO!" gene.

It should also be noted that an earlier study showed that low physical activity actually activated the FTO gene. So low activity makes it worse, and higher activity makes it go away. (This clearly aligns with my "You tell your body what to do" philosophy!)[9]

Now, can you even imagine if any of these study participants had employed the *REVVED* interval-based strength-training exercise plan? My belief is they would have further eradicated their genetic predisposition, possibly wiping it out, as the *REVVED* plan is not just about activity; it's about optimizing metabolism. Simple exercise doesn't really get the job done—much. As you will learn in chapter 7, exercise intensity is the often overlooked critical component of weight loss.[10]

My point is that as you age you may pick up a few pounds over what you once considered your "ideal" weight, but don't suddenly think that 50-plus pounds of additional fat is a result of genetics. It's not.

REVVED Component Number 3: Sleep

Sleep is an essential component of *REVVED* behavior, but most of us skimp on it. The American Cancer Society conducted a survey in 1960 and found that most Americans were sleeping 8 to almost 9 hours a night (that's me now, by the way). Then, in 1995, the National Sleep Foundation found that the number had dropped to 7 hours. Today, if you can believe it, more than 30 percent of adults report sleeping less than 6 hours a night.[11] That's a disaster, because sleep deprivation eradicates your *REVVED* goal of permanent weight loss.

Sleep Deprivation

Lack of sleep disrupts an almond-size part of your brain called the hypothalamic-pituitary-adrenal axis, or, for short, HPA. Basically, when you are sleep deprived, your hypothalamus assumes there is a problem and tells your pituitary gland, "Fix this." Your pituitary gland is a small endocrine organ that performs many functions, one of which is to monitor the production of hormones as they relate to muscle.[12] What has been found is that an "unhappy" hypothalamus tells the pituitary gland to produce the stress hormone cortisol. Cortisol has proven to be catabolic, meaning that it cannibalizes muscle.

Simply put, by skimping on sleep, you tell your body, "Houston, we have a problem," and it responds by producing cortisol and chewing up muscle. You *know* the human body is very smart. When you decide that you are going to "stay up and get one more thing done," your behavior dictates that you do just that, stay up. You are vehemently telling your brain and your body to get rid of muscle (that is, to decrease a *REVVED* metabolism), and it is listening.[13]

Here is the research to support this fact. Test subjects with an average age of between thirty-five and forty-nine and an average weight of 179 pounds were placed in two groups. One group had to be in bed for 8½ hours while the other had to be in bed for only 5½ hours. They stayed in the lab for fourteen days at a time, eating 1,450 calories a day; they were allowed to move around, but not to exercise. After three months, the study was repeated with the same subjects. Again, all subjects had to stay in the lab for fourteen days.

Since none of us falls asleep right away (except maybe me—the moment my head hits the pillow, I'm out), the "true" difference in sleep amounted to 2 hours and 11 minutes. Doesn't sound like much, does it?

But wait. At the end of this study, all participants lost about 14½ pounds eating 1,450 calories a day. Not bad. But when they examined what was lost, muscle or fat, the difference between the two groups was huge:

> The 8½-hour-a-night group lost 50 percent fat, 50 percent muscle, which makes sense since they didn't strength-train (you will lose *no* muscle on this plan, so this won't happen to you).

> The 5½-hour-a-night group lost 25 percent fat, 75 percent muscle, which shows that sleep deprivation, and the release of cortisol, is killing your muscle even more than just dieting alone.

When the study began, the average basal metabolic rate per participant was 2,140. By the end of the study:

> The 8½-hour group had dropped their basal metabolic rate to 1,505.

> The 5½-hour group had dropped their basal metabolic rate to 1,391.

Don't forget—all subjects ate the same 1,450 calories and had an identical amount of activity, but sleep deprivation made them lose even more muscle than fat. That's dreadful.

In addition to ridding your body of muscle, sleep deprivation also produces two detrimental hormonal effects that disrupt a *REVVED* metabolism. They are a reduction in the levels of leptin and an increase in those of ghrelin.

Leptin is a hormone that regulates both energy intake and energy expenditure, including appetite and metabolism. The role of leptin will pop up frequently in the *REVVED* weight-loss plan. Leptin was discovered by Jeffrey M. Friedman at Rockefeller University in 1994. Leptin is actually a protein

There is another body of research that shows that any calorie-restricted diet adhered to without strength training will eradicate 70 percent muscle and 30 percent fat. I didn't include this research because the percentages seemed high from what I have read and experienced with myself and my clients in the past. So, please know, for argument's sake, that I took the conservative side of research and said you lose 50 percent muscle and 50 percent fat. That may be the *best* you can do without strength training, and don't attempt any weight-loss plan while sleep deprived. You are better off doing nothing at all and just living at your present size until you are ready to tackle both a better sleep strategy and strength training. I mean that. *Don't* attempt any diet plan without strength training—ever. Don't worry though—I'm going to give you the perfect plan.

comprised of 167 amino acids, predominately manufactured in white fat (that's the vast majority of your body fat, remember), but also in brown fat (which you *want* on your body, as I explained earlier), the placenta, ovaries, skeletal muscle, stomach, mammary cells, bone marrow, pituitary gland, and liver.[14]

Leptin brings on the "I'm getting full" feeling. It does so by counteracting two potent feeding stimulators *and* promoting an appetite suppressant. That's why we like to have leptin circulating in our bodies. Sleep deprivation has been found to reduce leptin levels, and that reduction happens fast. The Wisconsin Sleep Cohort study showed that those who slept for 5 hours, in comparison to those that slept for 8, reduced leptin levels by 15.5 percent. That will absolutely result in your eating more and having less energy, and it will put the brakes on your *REVVED* goals.[15]

Here is a list of behaviors that optimize leptin production:

- **Eat a big, protein-rich breakfast first thing in the morning.** You will learn in chapter 4 that protein will always be included in your big breakfasts, as it helps trigger satiety mechanisms.

- **Cut out the white, as in the refined, simple carbs as well as sugars.** They are devoid of any nutrients and vitamins and are the true definition of "empty calories." They also cause an imbalance of your hormones, especially insulin. I have eliminated them in your 28-day *REVVED* Eating Plan and would urge you to avoid them forever.

- **Don't snack, because snacking keeps insulin and other hormones working when they should be resting.** I only have you eating a snack post-workout or when you know you will have more time in between meals than you should in order to avoid the blood sugar dips and subsequent hunger. Most diet plans include two or three snacks. I disagree. With three properly balanced meals you only need one snack, post-exercise. You will learn more about insulin and when to snack in chapter 4.

- **Lower the inflammation throughout your body.** Quick tip: Tea is amazing for lowering inflammation throughout your body, so you might brew up a cup right now as you are reading this book.[16]

Ghrelin is predominately a stomach-derived peptide that stimulates appetite. Similar to leptin, ghrelin will pop up again in subsequent chapters. Those of us on this *REV*olutionary diet plan don't like ghrelin, as it tells us to eat more. In the same Wisconsin Sleep Cohort study referenced for leptin, those who slept 5½ hours versus those who slept 8½ had ghrelin levels that were 14.9 percent higher.

A very similar study on sleep deprivation and its effect on ghrelin and leptin was conducted at the University of Chicago Clinical Research Center with twelve healthy young men. Once again, sleep deprivation:

Decreased leptin by 18 percent

Increased ghrelin by 28 percent

Increased hunger, or the physical feeling your body experiences when it needs food, by 24 percent

Increased appetite, or the desire to eat, which is sometimes triggered by hunger but more often stimulated by cravings, habits, availability of food, emotions, and boredom, to name a few, by 23 percent[17]

Please note that the 23 percent appetite increase referenced above included higher cravings for calorie-dense foods with high carbohydrate content, which you just learned will also diminish leptin levels. Sounds like a chips-pizza-cookie party to me.

Nutrition researcher Steven Heymsfield, of Columbia University, states: "When you haven't had a lot of sleep, your body reacts much the same as if you haven't eaten enough. These hormonal changes also seem to signal the body to put the brakes on metabolism and cling to fat stores more tenaciously."[18] Sounds to me like a *REV*elation that you must get more sleep!

Please note, too much dieting also inhibits leptin levels. That is why I continually say *don't* diet if you're not going to eat a high-protein breakfast, get appropriate sleep, minimize stress, and strength-train with intensity.

Repeated dieting makes hormonal matters worse. That's why I finally put this fully comprehensive plan together. It provides the total sum of what leads to a lean lifestyle forever. Plus, the plunging leptin levels experienced by those who are sleep deprived and stressed only lead us to the enemy: hunger. You will read all about my take on hunger in chapter 4.

But wait—there are three more hormones that are strongly affected by lack of sleep:

1. **Insulin.** A University of Chicago Medical Center study showed that after just six nights of only 4 hours of sleep each, the insulin and blood-glucose levels of participants were so significantly impaired that they were nearing a prediabetic state. If you can believe it, after just one night of 4 hours of sleep, many of those in the study had blood-sugar panels similar to those with type 2 diabetes.[19]

2. **Cortisol.** This stress hormone also immediately spikes as a result of sleep deprivation. Again, the body thinks, "There must be some danger, because I am not asleep, and I must prepare for that danger." As you know, cortisol cripples a *REVVED* metabolism, so you need to do everything in your power to minimize or eliminate it, except when it is really needed, which is rare.

3. **Testosterone.** This hormone is essential for muscle growth (you should *love* that, because muscle is the engine of your newfound *REVVED* body), increased metabolism (*REVVED* again), sex drive, and pumping energy. Skimp on sleep and you skimp on all the powerful *REVVED*-up benefits of testosterone. Oh, and the interval-based strength training I will teach you in chapter 7 boosts testosterone for both men *and* women, as we both need it. Testosterone tends to decline with age, so let's put the brakes on that and adopt *REVVED* behaviors that increase it as much as possible.

Do You Need More of Better Sleep?

First you need to stop the "I really don't need that much sleep" or "I'm just going to stay up and get one more thing done" thinking. Yes, you do need more sleep. What I find is that feeling lethargic and tired all the time becomes your "new normal." It's not a positive "new normal" (like your new, lighter, leaner body will be once it's *REVVED* up). This is a negative one, and you may be so used to this feeling that you have forgotten what it's like to be energized and productive. When you stay up to get "one more thing done," you all but guarantee that you won't be very productive the next day, because you will be sleep deprived.

When you get past your old belief system, then you start new *REVVED* behaviors that will enhance both the quality and quantity of your sleep. You need to develop what I call a "sleep strategy" to get 7 to 8 hours of quality sleep a night.

Start by determining the following:

1. **What time are you going to get up tomorrow morning?** If the answer is 6:00 A.M., then you need to count backward to the time you should go to bed tonight to achieve that 7 to 8 hour *sweet* spot. The answer to that would be sometime between 9:30 and 10:00 P.M., and that doesn't mean thinking about it at 11:00. You start actively thinking about it at 9:00 and begin the toothbrushing—plus flossing (a *REVVED* behavior, as it reduces inflammation)—and other nighttime rituals that tell your mind and body, "We are soon going to sleep."

2. **What else are you going to do before you go to bed?** Choose one of the following, and the odds increase that you will quickly fall asleep:

   a. **Take a warm bath—relax!** Put your body in the parasympathetic relaxation mode, which I will explain in the next chapter. For now, know that it's the "calm" state of being and the opposite of stress.

   b. **Light scented candles.** Lavender, chamomile, and ylang-ylang are popular sleep inducers.

   c. **Reduce the lights in your bedroom.** Tell your mind and body that it's time to go to bed. When it gets dark out or you dim the lights, this optimizes the body's production of melatonin. Melatonin is a hormone produced in the pineal gland that plays a starring role in your sleeping and waking cycle, also known as your circadian rhythm. Melatonin starts to increase in the early evening and is at its peak while you are sleeping, then drops off prior to your waking up. Again, reducing the light in your room helps produce this powerful, beneficial hormone.

   d. **Cool down your room.** The optimal body temperature for sleep is between 60 and 80 degrees. A decrease in your core temperature actually initiates sleepiness and the production of melatonin. Therefore, artificially creating a cooler sleep environment will result in falling asleep faster and staying asleep longer.

e. **"Reach out and touch someone."** Yes, there are powerful benefits from human contact, which include the release of oxytocin, which you can get from just hugging and touching, and even more so from, um, "finishing." This will help you sleep better that night and reduce stress for days afterwards. Oh, and it burns calories. (*Note:* You don't even have to "reach out and touch someone." You may elect to simply "reach out and touch" yourself, and that can be as simple as rubbing a body oil or lotion on your hands, arms, shoulders, abdomen, legs, and feet, or you can get more creative. I'll leave that up to you.)

3. **What you are *not* going to do before bed.** Here are some points:

   a. **No pets in the bed, ever.** The Mayo Clinic says that 53 percent of pet owners with pets in the bed reported sleep disruption.[20] Ditto for the kids, as I know when my son crawls into bed with me, he kicks me in the head all night. He also sleeps on a diagonal. I have a king-size bed, and even then, with him in there, I'm huddled up in a fetus-like ball. Not the most restful way to sleep.

   b. **Limit late-night exercise.** The general rule is that you should stop exercising at least 3 hours before the time you plan to go to bed. Exercise stimulates you, which may make it harder for you to wind down.

   c. **Restrict caffeine after noon.** Some people are able to drink or eat foods containing caffeine later in the day, while others are more sensitive and those drinks or foods disrupt their ability to fall asleep. Do your own research, and figure out what works for you. Did quitting caffeine by noon help you fall asleep faster that night? If so, you might make that a new *REVVED* behavior, or experiment with cutting caffeine out entirely.

   d. **Curb your alcohol consumption.** Alcohol may disrupt your sleep depending on the following:

      - **How much you drank that night.**

      - **How much you generally drink, which affects the extent to which alcohol enables you to fall asleep faster.** Those who consume alcohol infrequently do find that the alcohol acts as a sedative and allows them to fall asleep faster. Those who drink more frequently, as in almost nightly, may find that more and more alcohol is required to achieve the same sedative results; the excessive alcohol then disrupts the second half of a full night's sleep. Excessive alcohol results in you waking up and clearly not feeling well rested even if the recommended duration, 7 to 8 hours, was achieved.

- **What time you drank.** The alcohol most damaging to the quality of sleep is that consumed very close to bedtime, whereas drinking at "happy hour" or with an early dinner may not contribute to any sleepless or less restful nights.

- **What you ate with your alcohol.** Consuming alcohol on an empty stomach or after eating very little may result in a higher blood-alcohol level, which, once again, may enable you to fall asleep fast, but then result in your waking up frequently followed by difficulty falling back asleep.

> To supplement with melatonin or not to supplement, that is the question. Some studies point to melatonin's effectiveness with regard to falling asleep faster for those who struggle with it. It's also beneficial for people who work the night shift, and therefore need to sleep during the day, and for the blind, who don't have the benefit of experiencing the light of day. I have had clients who swear by their melatonin when they travel overseas or through various time zones. First follow all my instructions in this chapter before considering a melatonin supplement, and then consult with your doctor before taking one. Please note that there are other benefits of melatonin, such as helping cancer patients extend their lives, guarding the nervous system against degenerative disease, such as stroke and Alzheimer's disease, preventing migraines, reducing anxiety before surgery, and even quitting smoking.

As I said, it has been found that small amounts of alcohol may actually help you fall asleep faster. They have also been found to increase slow-wave sleep, which is the deep state of sleep that allows the brain and body to recover and allows the secretion of the essential *REVVED* growth hormone (much more on growth hormone later on). Slow-wave sleep also strengthens immunity, promotes healing and regeneration of bones, muscles, and other tissue, and accounts for approximately 75 to 80 percent of the time you are asleep.

When you perform the *REVVED* Exercise Plan, you will understand that it's all about creating microscopic tears in your muscles through strength training. Please don't think creating microscopic tears is a negative. It is not.

It's a very big positive to the exercise plan. After creating the tears, the rebuilding process begins, which is essential to your reshaped, *REVVED*-up, lean body, so increasing slow-wave sleep (when this rebuilding takes place) is a plus.

Unfortunately, too much booze:

1. Disrupts REM sleep, which is when memory and concentration are enhanced for the following and future days. REM stands for rapid eye movement, which occur during this form of sleep, as opposed to the slow-wave sleep just discussed. REM typically accounts for between 20 and 25 percent of a night's sleep. It is also the time when most of our dreaming occurs. Alcohol pushes REM sleep aside (because of the sedative effect) and heads us directly into slow-wave sleep. Then, as the effects of the alcohol wear off, the body attempts to make up for the lost REM sleep, and we may wake up sweating, feeling anxious, or having nightmares. Because the body is stressed from not following a more normal REM/slow-wave cycle, the nature of the dreams becomes more vivid and stressful, which translates to nightmares.

2. Causes us to have to get up and go to the bathroom multiple times, since alcohol acts like a diuretic and flushes fluid out of the body.

3. Exacerbates sleep apnea for those who already suffer from that sleep-altering, stress-inducing physical issue.

4. Reacts poorly with both natural and prescription sleep aids, as it may make them far more potent and dangerous. Please don't combine alcohol with any type of sleep aid.

On a final note, women have been found to metabolize alcohol faster than men. This means they get hit harder when they start to drink, so pace yourself to stay within the 4-ounce recommendation for enhanced health. If you are in a social setting where you know you will honestly consume more than that, make sure to include more protein before drinking, because protein stays in your stomach longer (more on that in chapter 4) and will slow the absorption of the alcohol. Also, studies have found that women get up more often in the night, stay awake longer, and actually sleep fewer hours after they drink alcohol than they would have had they abstained.

Gentlemen, I hear from my clients all the time, that when you drink, your snoring gets *loud*. Similar to what happens to those with sleep apnea, the relaxation decreases muscle tone in the upper airway. That causes the usual level of snoring to increase and potentially disturb your sleep *and* the restful sleep of those within earshot.[21]

Interestingly enough, what you do first thing in the morning will help to optimize sleep that night. Again, your goal is to tell your body what you want it to do and to get your sleeping and waking cycle primarily under your control. As I said in the introduction, the more you give consistent cues to your body, the more it will respond in a positive way.

So, first thing in the morning, I want you to reverse many of the behaviors I urged you to do at night. Now we want you *REVVED* up. Therefore you should do the following:

1. **Take your usual shower, but at the end play the "cold shower" game.** Start turning the water temperature down. No, it doesn't have to be freezing cold like when your water heater broke down. Just make it cold*er*. We have ten to twenty times the receptors for cold than we have for warm. Remember when you were a kid how refreshing it was to jump into a cool pool on a hot summer day? What about running through a sprinkler? That's the same concept. By giving your body a jolt, you actually tell it, "Yep, we're up and on and going to be productive and energized," and cold water accomplishes that miraculously.

2. **Turn on the lights.** Open up the drapes for natural light. Take your coffee or tea outside. Let the sunshine beat on you for a few minutes. Light wakes your body up and, similar to the "coldish" shower, tells your mind and your body that it's time to spring into action. I also think it's a great way to start your day. Plus, giving the clear "light" message "we are up and on" will help you later at night to fall asleep. Pushing the "on" button so strongly causes the body to think later in the day, "I'm going to have to get a good night's sleep because I bet I'm going to be asked to be 'on' again early tomorrow morning, and I want to be ready." Once again, behavior drives your body's response, both positively and negatively.

One simple way to know you are optimizing your sleeping and waking cycle is to get up each morning without an alarm clock. When I am at home, I set an alarm every night, probably out of fear of oversleeping, but almost never need it. I get aggravated when I'm making breakfast, hear its signal, and have to run into my bedroom to turn it off. But I do love the fact that my body knows what time it is supposed to get up. It knows because I told

Interestingly, cold has been shown to help activate the brown fat in the body. Here is some research to back it up: "A NASA scientist told *ABC News* that in studying the effects of temperature on astronauts, he saw people's metabolism boost by 20 percent in environments as mild as 60 degrees. A Joslin researcher told National Public Radio that 3 ounces of brown fat could burn 400 to 500 calories daily."[22]

Therefore, taking a cold*er* shower in the morning may both help optimize your circadian rhythm, so you fall asleep faster and activate your brown fat, and boost your metabolism and calorie burn. Don't torture yourself. Just go through your usual routine, but at the end of the shower, start to turn the temperature down. I would say the lower you go, the more benefit you may derive, but that's just my opinion.

One more point: I have actually opened Chicago's first cryotherapy treatment center, called Chicago CryoSpa. Cryotherapy is a cold-therapy experience that occurs in a cryo-sauna, where you stand for 2 to 3 minutes to shock your body with cold, or with a nitrogen gas stream that comes out of a piece of equipment called the "elephant," since the wand dispensing the stream resembles an elephant's trunk.

Both applications help to

Repair muscles and joints

Rebuild collagen, which forms the building blocks of our skin, tendons, and ligaments

Reduce inflammation (more on inflammation later)

Achieve a *REVVED*-up brain (Those who suffer from depression have found considerable benefit from the endorphin release.)

Activate your brown fat, warm you back up, and boost your metabolism (That is clearly going to *burn* though a lot of calories.)

A cryo spa may be coming to your city in the near future, but they are already in Los Angeles, Atlanta, and Minneapolis, to name a few. Just know cold therapy, such as the cold shower I recommended, does a great deal to promote muscle-tissue healing to optimize the *REVVED* Exercise Plan and to activate brown fat to boost calorie burn.

it what I wanted it to do. Part of that "telling" came from going to bed at around the same time each night.

One more *REVVED* sleep strategy is to aim to go to bed and get up at the same times, within 30 minutes, each night and day. That "signal" tells your body when it should wind down and when it should be *REVVED* up. Once again, the body loves patterns. You will see that theme prevail through this plan. Start with one of the most essential components, which is sleep. Tell your body when you need it to be on and when it can slow down and ultimately turn off. It will thank you with optimal energy, optimal brainpower, and the optimal *REVVED*-up metabolism. Why do we go back to the same restaurants or resorts? We do so because we loved the experience, the food, the ambiance, the service, and we know what to expect. Your mind and your body work the same way. Give them what they want regularly, meet expectations, and they will keep coming back with more and more of the best they have to offer.

Recovery Sleep

Can you make up for sleep deprivation on the weekends? This is known as "recovery" sleep. Most research simply states that it's better to have made up for the lost sleep over the weekend (or whenever you can) rather than living in a chronically sleep-deprived state. One particular study proved that the brain actually knows it has been sleep deprived, so it enables you to sleep both longer and deeper when given the opportunity.[23] Although it is not the perfect solution, most participants in this study reported that one good *long* (around 10-hour) sleep helped them feel closer to normal the first morning. It took a second night of recovery sleep or even a good long nap after the first night of recovery sleep to enable them to feel themselves the second morning. Is it an ideal strategy? Probably not, as the days you really needed optimal brain functioning were most likely during the week. With this "recovery" behavior, you're pretty wiped out on the weekdays but more alert on the weekends.[24]

Another strategy is called "banking sleep" when you know, in advance, that you are going to be sleep deprived. If you have to travel overseas and don't sleep well on planes, then a *REVVED* behavior would be to guarantee that you "bank up" the night before and sleep 8-plus hours. Please note, if you have a stressful day ahead of you and you know it in advance, make it a priority to get to bed early the night before. That way you will think more clearly, have increased energy, and simply be better prepared to deal with any challenging situation.

To nap or not to nap when it comes to sleep deprivation? That really depends on timing and duration of the nap. A daily "scheduled" nap will play into your body's circadian rhythm, or the sleeping and waking cycle, that I introduced you to earlier in this chapter. It goes back to the "routine" that our body loves when it comes to so many behaviors, including sleep. Recall what I said about babies. They *love* to nap at the same time each day, whether it is once or twice.

The same goes for you. You might plan, each and every day around 3:00 P.M. (or whenever is best for you), to put your head down for a nap. Obviously, many of us have work environments where there isn't any opportunity for a nap, but think about where you might be able to take a break that might include one. Even 10 minutes of nap time can be beneficial to the body.

Here's the research on the amount of time you need to nap:

1. Ten to 20 minutes is the "gold standard" if your goal is increased energy and alertness. I'm a fan of this type of nap, as afterwards I just jump right back up into action with little to no grogginess. That occurs because I stayed in a light sleep.

2. A 30-minute nap may not make sense, because you increase the risk of getting up feeling groggy. Researchers call that "sleep inertia." It might be best to cut the nap off at 20 minutes.

3. If you are napping to improve memory and have to go to a meeting or party and remember faces, names, and facts, go for an hour. You are going to hit some slow-wave sleep, which will cause the sleep inertia similar to the 30-minute nap, but the trade-off may be worth it and outweigh the benefits.

4. Oddly, a 90-minute nap that includes a full sleep cycle (lighter, deeper, and REM sleep) does not cause as much sleep inertia as the 30- to 60-minute choice, but it does significantly increase memory and creativity.[25]

I bet you never thought about why you were going to take a nap, what you were trying to accomplish, or planning the time of the nap in advance. You never did that because you were so sleep deprived that you just put your head down and was out or fell asleep in your chair unexpectedly. No plan and no consistency, which I have told you repeatedly your body loves. Nope, just a plain old "I'm exhausted" plop-down nap.

I hope that some of this research has convinced you to make your sleep habits a true contributor to the metabolism makeover you will achieve with the *REVVED* program. Actually, it is an essential part of the program, because this program has been formulated considering the benefits of each component. Being sleep deprived while attempting to lose weight will result in: muscle loss and ultimately weight gain.

The belief that you must get adequate sleep each night and, if not, at *least* schedule a nap—and subsequent follow-through behavior—will power your *REVVED*-up odds of successful, permanent weight loss.[26]

REVVED Component Number 4: Stress

REVVED **Fiction**   "You have a handle on how to manage your stress."

REVVED **Fact**   Stress slams a *REVVED* metabolism—hard!

I just told you that sleep deprivation increases the production of cortisol, the stress hormone, and that cortisol has been proven to be catabolic. We therefore have to believe that:

Sleep Down = Cortisol Up = Muscle *REVVED* Down

If we eliminate the sleep component, will *any* increase in cortisol production result in muscle and a *REVVED* reduction?

According to the Mayo Clinic, the stress response begins when a tiny region in the base of your brain sets off an alarm system in your body: "Through a combination of nerve and hormonal signals, this system prompts your adrenal glands, located atop your kidneys, to release a surge of hormones, including adrenaline and cortisol. Cortisol, the primary stress hormone, increases sugars (glucose) in the bloodstream, enhances your brain's use of glucose, and increases the availability of substances that repair tissues. Cortisol also curbs functions that would be nonessential or detrimental in a fight-or-flight situation. It alters immune system responses and suppresses the digestive system, the reproductive system, and growth processes."[27]

That last line—suppresses growth processes—should be the one that causes you to pause, because it includes chewing up your precious muscle and/or preventing the growth of muscle as it responds to interval-based strength training. This clearly inhibits your *REVVED* behaviors, such as strength training, which require growth processes to spring into action. Chronic stress is to a *REVVED* metabolism what kryptonite was to Superman!

I'm also convinced, and will prove to you in subsequent chapters, that the high production of insulin, a storage hormone, is causing your body to store more fat. The second sentence said cortisol "increases sugars (glucose) in the bloodstream." Insulin, as you will soon learn, will have to be released to get the sugar to where it can either go to work or go to bed, that is, store itself as body fat. More often than not, it's the former rather than the latter, but I will give you a full discussion of insulin in chapter 4.

Now, periodic stress is part of all of our lives and does not deserve a bad rap. Back in prehistoric days, predominately men would be walking in the wild looking for dinner, as their families only "ate what they killed." Say you are a prehistoric hunter foraging around, spear firmly over your shoulder, and you came upon a tiger, who decides that you looked tasty. To keep from becoming his midday meal, the stress (fight-or-flight) response kicks in, dumps glucose into your bloodstream for a burst of energy, and enables you to run like hell. It also accelerates your breathing, decreases your pain, and increases your immunity. Sounds good if you want to stay alive.

Then, once the threat of being eaten has passed, the body returns to its normal, relaxed "prethreat" state, called the parasympathetic response. The stress was there when you needed it and then disappeared when you didn't. Think of the stress response as the gas pedal and the relaxation, or parasympathetic response, as the brake. Both are valuable, so let's not say *all* stress is bad.

Chronic stress occurs when you live on the gas, pumping it down dozens, maybe hundreds of times a day, and lay off the brake completely. You never allow the body to return to its relaxed state. Cortisol levels remain high. In essence, you "blow out" the stress response's ability to adjust to situations and circumstances, and it simply stays turned on all the time. The body says, "If you are going to live on the gas pedal, then I'm going to just floor it." You therefore exist through most waking hours and, most likely, sleeping hours in an elevated "stressed-out" state. Although this results in a slew of negative effects, for our discussion it is important to know that the cortisol associated with stress is chewing up muscle while storing body fat in your midsection. It usually causes depression and sleep deprivation—the latter of which has clearly been found to lead to weight *gain*. You are also continually flooding your body with sugar and insulin. You are telling your body, "Store fat, store fat," and it's listening.

You know if you are stressed. You also probably don't appreciate it when people say, in a patronizing way, "Just try to relax." Right! I find you have to use specific stress-relieving strategies, and they include the following.

The Power of Breath

Deep breathing is a powerful antistress behavior. Just start with the belief "If I take deep breaths my stress hormone, cortisol, will go down," because that's a fact. Then follow that up with the *REVVED* behavior—deep breathing—and you've made a smart choice.

REVVED Fiction   "A breath is a breath is a breath."

REVVED Fact   Our most critical source of energy is oxygen.

Think of what it's like to watch a baby sleeping. You see the body expand before your very eyes as the child takes, long, deep, oxygenating (calming) breaths. They are long inhales, followed by equally long exhales. If only we would all continue to breathe like babies throughout our entire lives!

Instead, with age we start to take shorter breaths. By adulthood, we are taking fifteen to twenty breaths per minute, which is called "shallow" breathing. It doesn't sound like that big of a deal, but it is. That shallow breathing is an indication to our very smart brain that there is danger and we must be in fight-or-flight mode, the stress response. So, as with any stress, cortisol is pumped out. I've made it perfectly clear that cortisol is to a *REVVED* body what the bucket of water was to the Wicked Witch of the West—it dissolves it!

Our lungs are capable of holding two pints of air, but we rarely get in those two full pints and generally get in no more than one. We don't get the full two pints because we keep old, stale air trapped in our lungs because of shallow breathing.

There are problems with both how we are inhaling and exhaling. Ideally, you want

- a full, deep inhale, which brings oxygen to your blood,

followed by

- a full, rich exhale, to rid your body of carbon dioxide.

Not doing so actually puts the body in the fight-or-flight stress mode, and I think I have made it abundantly clear what stress does to your *REVVED* metabolism.

You may also remember that one of the characteristics of the stress response is quick, shallow breaths. By doing so, you just keep flashing a big sign, "Stress approaching, stress approaching," and your smart body prepares for the stress that never ends up coming. It stays in that "pedal to the floor" mode because you told it to. Don't do that.

When I give speeches, I almost always include the following information on deep breathing. It has been shown to:

1. **Reduce stress.** Researchers at West Virginia University noted that just 10 minutes a day of deep breathing—just 10 minutes—reduced stress by up to 44 percent.[28] That's a huge reduction for a 10-minute investment of your time, and definitely worth it in my opinion. I happen to do this all the time—and many times for more than 10 minutes.

   Here's the scenario. You're in traffic. You're running late. You're already irritated because your car is making that odd noise that you had checked, twice, and was told was nothing. You have a choice. You can hunch up your shoulders, jut out your chin, tense up your face, breathe shallowly, and make your stress hormones surge, which only throws gasoline on the flame. Or you can go to the breath. First, give yourself a quiet pep talk and say calmly, "There is nothing I can do about this situation now except to breathe deeply, calm down, and find a new car mechanic." You know which choice is the smart *REVVED* decision.

2. **Slow the growth of cancer cells.** Oncologists (cancer specialists) claim that cancer cells *cannot* flourish in a well-oxygenated environment. Translation: Breathe deeply. You also boost immunity, because it's impaired when the fight-or-flight response is first activated. Breathe deeply, put the brakes on chronic stress, return to the parasympathetic mode, and give yourself a big immunity boost. Visualize your immune function as a little Pac-Man, gobbling up antibodies, viruses, cancer cells—you name it. Remember when you were a kid and you kept going to the next level as you kept gobbling up the energy? Up the efficiency of your Pac-Man, and you all but guarantee a longer game and a longer life.

3. **Reduce caloric intake.** Sounds very *REVVED* to me! A study conducted at the University of Rhode Island found that mindful breathing in between bites helped participants reduce caloric intake by

10 percent. We all eat too fast. I know I did when I was struggling with my weight. Haven't you seen people wolf down their food in a few minutes—and I mean a few—and then reach for more? My take is that mindful breathing helps trigger satiety mechanisms, which is a core component of *REVVED* eating. You have to like that![29]

Breathing into Blackness

In my fourth book, *The 7-Day Energy Surge,* I introduced my readers to a method of breathing called "Breathing into Blackness." It has become such an essential part of my program that it had to become part of the *REVVED* plan.

This is a breathing exercise I'd like you to perform for at least 10 minutes a day. Ideally, you will do it with your eyes closed, but clearly that won't work well in the stressful traffic situation I used as an example. So you determine where and when it's best to allocate these 10 minutes. Just know I prefer it with your eyes shut and all lights off to optimize relaxation.

1. Position yourself sitting upright at your desk with your elbows on the top of the desk, or lie down on the floor.

2. Close your eyes and place the palms of your hands over your eyes with your fingertips resting on top of your head.

3. Relax all your other muscles, such as the neck and shoulders, as much as possible.

4. Expel all the stale, old, oxygen-free air out of your lungs by performing three big forced exhales.

5. Slowly begin to inhale through your nose. Ideally, you are going to inhale for six counts (this pace will be similar to what you are going to use when performing the *REVVED* Exercise Plan). It's one, one thousand, two, one thousand, three, one thousand, four, one thousand, five, one thousand, six, one thousand. Pause, then exhale through your mouth at the same speed. Visualize a straw in your mouth and you are exhaling through that small space.

6. Repeat this for 10 minutes.

7. As your body "destresses" and returns to the parasympathetic mode, you may notice your muscles relaxing. You may also notice that you are able to breathe in for more than the six counts. Go for it.

I try to start almost every day with this exercise. I don't get out of bed. I just lie there, after having woken without an alarm, and place one hand on my diaphragm and the other over both eyes to blacken the room out that much more. When I remember to, I grab a sleep mask from my bedside table and put that on. I then do this exercise for up to 10 minutes, and often I can get to ten counts on both the inhale and exhale.

I begin each morning relaxed, as I want a nice slow takeoff into the potential stresses of the day. Unfortunately, I find most people get up with an alarm blaring and have to slap the snooze button a minimum of three times, because they are so sleep deprived. Finally, they jolt upright, jump out of bed because they have overslept, and thus start the day totally stressed out. Cortisol is off and running, and they are pressing—hard—on the gas. Within minutes, they begin a process of flooring the car that lasts for the rest of the day. As you will learn throughout this book, what happens in the morning is key to metabolism. Your morning actions matter! You really need to take control of your morning liftoff, which sets the pace for your day.

It's like the difference between a rocket ship taking off and a jet taking off. The rocket ship takeoff begins with huge explosions, smoke, stairs and scaffolding falling away, more smoke, and more explosions; then it blasts upward. That's probably you.

Why not consider yourself the jet, as I do? Get into position on the runway with *REVVED* engines, start to move, and when you have hit airspeed, pull back and begin to take off. It's so smooth, so sexy. No explosions or jolts—just a lovely beginning of your journey of the day. Aim for that "jet takeoff."

I realize I can't immediately change the stresses you may be dealing with on a daily basis, such as kids, money, aging parents, a bad relationship, a demanding boss, needy friends—that's up to you. What I want to help you with is how you prepare yourself to respond to these situations and make them better. Are we striving for perfection (just another stress)? No. But let's at least have some plan of action.

Calming the Fat Away

"Calming the Fat Away" is the title of an article in the May 2012 issue of *O, The Oprah Magazine*, which I've both written for and been featured in. Researchers at the University of California at San Francisco were looking into a link between dangerous abdominal fat and thoughts about eating.

The goal of the study, according to lead author Jennifer Daubenmier, was to enable participants to "tune in to physical sensations of hunger, fullness and taste satisfaction and to eat based on that awareness" rather than the typical culprit—stress.

The training was basic. The forty-seven participants were taught to recognize negative feelings, including anger and anxiety, and then *not* turn to food, as they had in the past. After the four-month study, the results were impressive. The women who reported the *most* improvement in stress levels and subsequent mindful eating lost 4.2 ounces of belly fat. One participant lost as much as 25 ounces of belly fat, which is a lot. This was *all* done without dieting—just being more emotionally aware of what they were feeling, and not following the same eating pattern that they always had.

Here is the most interesting part of the study: All forty-seven participants experienced a drop in cortisol, which we know is that nasty hormone that chews up muscle and promotes belly fat. What I didn't know is that "fat cells in the abdomen have four times as many cortisol receptors as fat cells elsewhere; when you're under stress, cortisol binds to those cells and triggers them to store more fat."[30]

That must explain why there was such an impressive drop in belly fat of 4.2 ounces for the women who truly did report reduced stress and stress eating. We would expect some belly fat to be burned with more mindful, less caloric food choices, but this relationship between fat cells and cortisol had to explain the majority of the belly fat drop. That news made me think about certain friends who always appear stressed out and who have excess belly fat. Interesting.

I think all of us need to examine how food may be our "go to" solution when we are under stress.

One final thought: I subscribe to Paul "Ripples Guy" Wesselmann's e-mails, which come in every Monday. Fern DeLima, who helps run my world in the Chicago office, is a quintessential yoga-practicing hippie, but with a major type A perfectionist streak. She's great and gets a lot done. She urged me to sign up and just today, as I was literally finishing the book, this came to me from Paul:

> *I am so often encouraging you to think about what you could add to increase your effectiveness and enjoyment with work, school, and/or life. Today I invite you to be curious about stepping back, observing,*

and perhaps removing something (or someone?) from your life that no longer nourishes your spirit. Imagine a doctor calling back with results from recent lab work: "The good news is that everything looks fine; however, I think you should remove one or two projects from your full plate so you can maintain a proper balance and thrive for many years to come."

What might you remove, and what would it take to make the call?[31]

For the sake of having more calm in my life, I know I'm already thinking of what I should remove, and I urge you to do the same.

REVVED Component Number 5: Music

REVVED Fiction   "Music is just for entertainment."

REVVED Fact   Music fuels a *REVVED* metabolism.

Yes, music affects us!

Noted British researcher Sue Hallam tells us: "Music can influence our moods and some aspects of our behavior in ways that may be outside our conscious awareness. The fact that music is processed in many ways and has physical, emotional, and cognitive effects may be the key to its power."[32]

It's fascinating when you think that music possesses that much power. You have repeatedly read that stress dashes a *REVVED* metabolism. Calming music has the power to lower the heart rate and deepen the breath, both of which lead the body to the relaxation response. Powerful.

Numerous studies show that music therapy works to fight depression, and you don't even have to listen to music often. Researchers at the National University of Singapore examined a total of seventeen individual studies that proved listening to music as little as once a week can help beat the blues. There are various opinions about why music is beneficial, but it appears the following is true:

- Music helps distract us from depressing thoughts. For want of a better phrase, it appears to help us "take our mind off it" for a while.

- Music helps produce the feel-good hormone dopamine, which makes us feel excited.

- Music, especially songs that have a sad theme, help us feel that we are not alone. Knowing that there are others out there who also struggle with sad thoughts and feelings may reduce the "why me" anxiety.[33]

Frequently, anxiety and depression go hand in hand, and anxiety is going to put the body in the cortisol-infused, fight-or-flight stress mode. By putting on the brake, or placing the body in the parasympathetic relaxation state, the stress hormones, I believe, subside and with that a better feeling about oneself emerges. This is just my theory, but it makes perfect sense to me.

A study at Baltimore Hospital proved how powerful music can be. Some people received 10 milligrams of an anti-anxiety drug; others got no drug but listened to music. Both groups derived the same benefits.[34]

Equally powerful is music's effect on sleep. One study conducted at Case Western Reserve University showed that college students who listened to soothing music 45 minutes before bedtime had a slower breath rate, reported falling asleep faster, and recalled more vivid dreams in the morning."[35]

The majority of our dreams occur in REM sleep. REM plays a critically important role with regard to the mind, memory, and learning. I like to think of REM sleep as the ultimate computer-screen organizer. You know when you have too many files and folders on your computer desktop? Sometimes it's a mess. Mine is now as I am finishing this book and devoting all my energy to final edits. What if I told you that getting more sleep, and specifically more REM sleep, would do all the organizing for you? You would wake up with more clarity, and because your brain got organized, you would have to ability to make better decisions and choices. I would go as far as to say that getting more REM sleep actually makes you smarter. REM sleep also promotes the feel-good hormones such as dopamine and serotonin, so you are both smarter *and* happier. I will go so far as to say:

REM = Considerable *REVVED* Outcomes

Therefore, to build on the sleep strategy I introduced you to, you should listen to soothing music at night, and not just before going to bed. Listen to it all evening.

I come home and immediately put on soothing music, usually classical, but I'm also a big fan of movie scores by John Williams, who wrote the music for so many *huge* films. Google him. You will be shocked that so many of the most memorable scores are by him. As I write today, I'm switching between the soundtracks of *Sabrina*, *The Accidental Tourist*, and *Somewhere in Time*. If a movie puts me in a really good mood, listening to the music brings back the memories and makes me more relaxed, productive, and happy.

As beneficial as soothing music is in the evening, in the morning choose the exact opposite. Turn on your favorite *pounding* music. If you can, blast it all over the house. If you worry about disturbing others, pop in your earbuds, and listen while shaving, applying makeup, or preparing and eating your big breakfast. By all means sing along, because the breathing that occurs during singing reduces stress. This is just like throwing the lights on in the morning to tell the mind and body "Let's get up." You will start your day both happy and relaxed.

Music and Eating

Music also has the ability to determine the rate at which we eat and chew. Soothing music, such as classical music, conjures up images of elegance, beauty, and sophistication. With it, we eat more slowly, take longer pauses between bites as we place our silverware down, and relax. That's great. The opposite happens when we eat to up-tempo music. We actually start chewing to the beat, so don't have that kind of music on while you are eating unless your goal is weight gain.

Music and Exercise

The research conclusively shows that listening to music while exercising promotes endurance and, far more important (as you will soon learn), intensity. Costas Karageorghis, from London's Brunel University School of Sport and Education, is one of the leading authorities on the relationship between exercise and music. He actually says, "Music is like a legal drug for athletes." He finds that music can "reduce the perception of effort significantly and increase endurance by as much as 15 percent."[36] That a big increase from something as simple and accessible as music.

To be honest, the bulk of the research on music and exercise was conducted while participants performed classic cardiovascular exercise, something I never, ever want you to do, and I will give you the whole reason why in chapter 7. But there has also been some research on the effects music achieves when it comes to strength training. There was a very simple study done at York St. John University in the United Kingdom. The researchers asked students to simply hold a 2.4-pound weight straight out in front of their bodies. They were prompted to hold the weight at shoulder height. Just hold it, mind you, nothing more. Interestingly, while listening to powerful music with strong lyrics, they could hold the weight 10 percent longer.[37]

I am inconsolable when I forget my iPod or have not properly charged it and am getting ready to hit my strength training with gusto. I NEED music when I strength-train and know that it enables me to blast through those last essential repetitions (a *REVVED* behavior).

I strongly urge all of you to create your own favorite exercise music track and ideally set it up so that near the end of the workout, when you are just about done, your favorite songs come on to power you through those last reps. In fact, you can set up a playlist for each of your transitions throughout the day, so that you've already compiled music that fits your intention. *REVVED* actions should be intentional.

REVVED Component Number 6: The Thyroid

According to the Cleveland Clinic, "The thyroid is a small gland, shaped like a butterfly, that rests in the middle of the lower neck. Its primary function is to control the body's metabolism (the rate at which cells perform duties essential to living). To control metabolism, the thyroid produces hormones, T4 and T3, which tell the body's cells how much energy to use."[38]

At least 30 million Americans have a thyroid disorder, and half of them are undiagnosed, according to the American Association of Clinical Endocrinologists. If you are a woman over thirty-five, your odds of having the disorder are about 30 percent. That's high.[39]

What causes the thyroid malfunction? There could be a number of causes, including your genes, an autoimmune disease, stress, pregnancy, poor nutrition, or simply the toxins that you eat, drink, or breathe. To be honest, sometimes doctors just don't know.

When the thyroid produces too many hormones, a condition called hyperthyroidism, it frequently results in bulging eyes, a rapid heart rate, and weight loss. I know, you are probably saying you would love the weight loss, but hyperthyroidism causes many problems in the body and is not something to aspire to.

On the other hand, hypothyroidism, when the thyroid does not produce enough hormones, seriously depletes your *REVVED* metabolism. This may be an issue for some of you if you notice any of the following:

You struggle with low energy levels, as a low-functioning thyroid will make you feel lethargic.

You have slow-growing hair and nails, especially if there is a distinct change from the past. (Often hair stylists are the first to notice a change in hair texture or volume.)

You suddenly feel cold all the time. Some of my clients who complained about being cold all the time, more often than not, found out their thyroid was not functioning properly.

You suffer from constipation. If there has been a big change in your bowel movements, you may have a thyroid issue.

You have frequent headaches. And women suffer from headaches more frequently than men. According to Jennifer Kelly of the Atlanta Center for Behavioral Medicine, "Studies have shown that women are 50 percent more likely to suffer headaches." She goes on to say that "women are also two and a half times more likely to be struck by a migraine."[40] Once they are treated for hypothyroidism, patients frequently report that they feel more "sharp" and "productive" than before.

You experience irregular menstrual cycles or have difficulty getting pregnant, as the thyroid plays a role in ovulation.

You suffer from high cholesterol or high blood pressure, especially if there hasn't been a history of it in your family.

You feel depressed. The thyroid impacts the feel-good hormone serotonin, which is what most antidepressant medications attempt to increase.

You have no interest in sex, which may be a function of low thyroid combined with the way you feel about your body given weight gain, the physical pain of headaches, or decreased energy.

If you are experiencing any of these symptoms, I suggest you ask your internist to recommend an endocrinologist (a thyroid specialist) for further testing.

Dr. Regina P. Walker, both a friend and a client, is a specialist in thyroid disorders. She has successfully treated a number of my friends and clients.

Here is what she has to say on the issue of thyroid testing and why you have to perform more extensive testing and blood work to determine proper thyroid levels:

> The average family practitioner orders a screening test called a TSH (thyroid stimulating hormone), which is a hormone secreted from the pituitary gland (the master endocrine organ) in the brain. The problem with this test is that it only reflects the opinion of the pituitary gland. By that I mean that it is a very good measure of change, so if we remove the thyroid surgically or destroy its function with radioactive iodine for Graves' disease, then the pituitary gland notes the drop in thyroid hormone levels in the bloodstream and the TSH increases in an attempt to get the thyroid gland to produce more thyroid hormone for the body. The pituitary gland does not know that the thyroid was removed or destroyed, so it will keep increasing the TSH level in attempts to get more thyroid hormone for the body to live on. Thus the problem is that if you lose your metabolism slowly, you have to lose almost 50 percent of your function before the TSH starts to go up to a level that would suggest to the family doctor that there is a problem.
>
> Now, if you measure the active thyroid hormones, Free T4 and Free T3, then you see how much thyroid hormone the patient actually is living on. So I get a Free T4 and Free T3 and a TSH to check the patient's current thyroid function, I get thyroid peroxidase antibodies and thyroglobulin antibodies to check for autoimmune disease, and finally I get a thyroglobulin level. All patients also get an ultrasound of the thyroid gland, so we can see the size and texture of the gland, and we also can determine if there are nodules (circular areas in the thyroid that can represent tumors, benign or malignant).
>
> With regard to good levels to live at, that is a hard question to answer because optimal levels are based on so many factors. Good levels for an individual are determined by the patient's age, gender, previous thyroid function (i.e., if a patient had a thyroidectomy), anxiety levels, and cardiac history. So there are really many factors that have to be considered before an optimal level can be decided upon. It is really best for patients to find a doctor who is knowledgeable in the thyroid world to work with.

From my experience with clients and medication, I know that some thyroid specialists err on the conservative side, as in prescribing less medication, while others are willing to be more aggressive in pushing the thyroid to the high side of acceptable. That is something you should be aware of when interviewing a specialist for treatment.

I bet many of you were surprised by the word "interview" when seeing your doctor. Just as I said in the introduction, you are the captain of your own ship. Don't just go to any doctor—go to the one you feel is the best person for the job, as he or she will be the navigator of your ship, your health, and your *REVVED* outcome.

REVVED Component Number 7: Human Growth Hormone

By the time you hit middle age, at around forty, you have lost 80 percent of your growth hormone. Every year after that, you lose 2 percent. Human growth hormone (HGH), which is secreted by the pituitary gland, serves a number of vital functions, including the following:

Keeping you young and lean

Maintaining metabolism, as in keeping it up and running and not diminishing as much with age (FYI, the best way we enable the body to accomplish this goal is by following the *REVVED* Exercise Plan.)

Strengthening your bones, skin, and muscles (the engine of *REVVED*)

Tightening your skin

Promoting rapid hair and nail growth

Decreasing fat accumulation

Improving circulation

Creating a more favorable cholesterol profile

Protecting your organs from aging[41]

To make HGH, to compensate for what you lose with aging, you need the following:

1. **Strength training.** As you will learn in chapter 7, strength training must be done with intensity and heavy resistance in order for you to derive optimal benefits. You create microscopic tears in your muscles when you strength-train with intensity, and repairing

them requires human growth hormone. Plus, HGH stimulates the growth of new muscle fibers and causes the release of fat.[42] *All* good for a *REVVED* body.

2. **High-intensity interval training, often referred to as HIT.** The goal is to push your heart rate above what is termed your anaerobic threshold, which in lay terms means you are working at such a high intensity that you are getting out of breath and are probably unable to comfortably speak. You should push your body to stay at this level for about 30 to 60 seconds and repeat it five times in your workout. This is what we will be doing at the end of the *REVVED* Exercise Plan. *Note:* Not only does the high-intensity interval training increase your human growth hormone but it also puts your feel-good, happy hormones into overdrive. You finish your workout with *more* energy than when you started.

3. **Clean, nutritious foods.** Cut out the quick empty carbs, because the big rush of glucose (which I will discuss in chapter 4) leads to a big release of insulin. Insulin inhibits human growth hormone's flow into the bloodstream, so we only want to call upon insulin when needed and only in an acceptable amount. Remember, stress dumps glucose into your bloodstream for added energy to run from the tiger (the stress). So since stress also causes a chain-reaction rush of insulin, you could connect the dots and say that stress also inhibits human growth hormone. (If it sounds like I'm "down on stress," I am!)

4. **Deep sleep.** Optimal growth hormone is produced in the deep stages of sleep. Therefore, the sleep strategy I introduced you to earlier becomes even more essential, because you want to complete as many full sleep cycles as possible to optimize human growth hormone. Since a 90-minute nap takes you through all the stages of a cycle, having a 90-minute nap will also enhance HGH. (Don't eat for about 2 hours before going to sleep, or the insulin released could inhibit human growth hormone's flow into the bloodstream.)

5. **Amino acids.** A protein-rich diet, which is what you will be consuming on your *REVVED* Eating Plan, is packed with amino acids. But there are certain specific amino acids that enable you to produce human growth hormone. In this instance, I recommend supplementing with a GOAL combination pill that contains the following:

a. **Glycine,** which builds muscle, promotes sleep, and is found in protein-rich foods, such as meat, fish, dairy, and legumes (though it is still best to supplement).

b. **Ornithine,** which helps with athletic performance, fatigue, and the efficiency of energy consumption. It has to be consumed as a supplement.

c. **Arginine,** which changes into nitric oxide in the body, is a neurotransmitter that improves circulation, helps blood vessels relax, and therefore regulates blood pressure. Although you should still supplement, arginine is found in red meat, fish, poultry, grains, nuts, seeds, and dairy products.

d. **Lysine,** which helps convert fatty acids to energy, lowers cholesterol, and aids the body's absorption of calcium for bone health. It also helps promote collagen growth, which is great for maintaining youthful skin (FYI, looking good is a *REVVED* benefit and therefore motivating for compliance to the plan). Foods containing lysine include red meat, pork, poultry, Parmesan cheese, cod, sardines, nuts, eggs, soybeans, dairy products, and legumes. Still, it is recommended that you supplement to achieve the increased production of HGH.

Women, don't ever worry about getting too big from strength training. It's impossible. You don't produce enough growth hormone or testosterone for that to ever happen. Strength training is *magic* on a woman's body. If you don't believe me, believe Jane Brody, a longtime health columnist for the *New York Times* who has repeatedly written, "Strength training makes women shrink and gives them a tiny physique." Go, Jane!

Or better yet, watch *ABC News* and get a look at Diane Sawyer. Diane is in the second half of her sixties. Does she look big? Bulky? Man-like? No, she looks elegant, lean, long, and (I've always been a stickler about posture) notice how she sits up. That's what happens when you listen to me and embrace an intense strength-training program. Go, Diane!

The Dr. Oz Show, which I've been on a number of times (he's a great, hard-working guy), really pushed this point home in a series of shows on energy and the benefits of producing more human growth hormone. He cited research from the University of Pittsburg that stated that supplementation can increase HGH production by 600 percent. The moment I read this research, I ran out and bought a bottle of supplements containing all four GOAL components at my neighborhood health-food store, so I'm performing my own research study. I'll keep you posted. Prepare to see the benefits when I look younger the next time you see me on television!

3

The REVelation

You are killing your metabolism with most diets, especially cleanses!

I know this chapter is going to get some of you riled up—and not in a good way. Some of you will staunchly disagree with me, because you love to cleanse over and over and over again. I firmly believe that this is something you should never, ever do, and you will soon learn why. But bring on the debate, as my goal is that you finally and fully understand why you keep losing weight and then gaining it back.

Classic Calorie-Reduced Diets

To lose weight, you have to go back to the balance-of-energy equation:

Calories In (Food & Drink) − Calories Out (AMR) = Your Current Body Weight

As I said earlier, some weight-loss experts disagree with this equation. They will tell you that the "quality" of calories matters more than the actual calories. They will say that the way protein is metabolized is different than the way white, processed carbs are metabolized. I agree with some of these points—the *REVVED* Eating Plan is filled with "quality" calories, and I do urge you to shun the white, processed carbs. But once they are metabolized differently, as a result of the hormonal response, they still function as a calorie, or unit of energy. Oops, looks like it's once again a numbers game—calories in minus calories out.

Now, you know I dislike the expression "losing weight," as to simply lose weight truly isn't your goal. Your goal is to lose fat. We saw in the previous chapter how two groups of people consuming 1,450 calories a day lost fat *and* muscle, because they didn't perform strength training. It's a fact, but muscle loss is not inevitable, and I will teach you how to *REV*erse that trend, adopt all the corrective behaviors, lose *all* fat . . . and then keep it off.

Let me be clear: It's all but impossible to keep the weight off on a traditional, calorie-restricted diet, as the vast majority of these unsuccessful plans rid your body of water, something you never want to do. The scale goes down, but you don't lose an ounce of fat. You just lose water from your cells, mostly by eliminating carbohydrates. Think of your cells as sponges full of water. When you eliminate the majority of carbohydrates, you wring the water out of the cells, and the scale goes down. Did you lose fat? Nope. And the moment you eat some carbohydrates, the "good" water weight comes back and the scale pops back up. We don't want to lose water. We need it, as you will learn, to fuel up the body's ability to burn fat for fuel, so don't do this to your body, because it will start to throw everything—your body's total balance, hormones, weight, fat, you name it—out of whack.

Then, as we just saw from the research in the last chapter, pure calorie-restricted diets rid the body of its long, lean, calorie-burning muscle. Once again, muscle is the engine of a *REVVED* metabolism, and losing it is devastating to your long-term weight-loss plans. You must practice all the *REVVED* behaviors to guarantee that you preserve and gain muscle at all times.

I'm always appalled by diets that don't include behaviors such as eating breakfast, progressive strength-training (I will explain the "progressive" part in chapter 7), a successful sleep strategy, and stress relief. They're ineffective and unethical.

Why do some authors do that? It's because they are giving their readers what they want to hear: "Don't exercise, skip breakfast, sleep as little as you like, and remember, raging stress is just a fact of life." First of all, only 54.7 percent of Americans exercised in August 2012.[1] While that number is up from the previous year, I bet 98 percent or more of those people are just walking for exercise. Walking falls into the category of what I refer to as "active rest." Sure, it will help you to reduce your risk of disease, such as heart attack, stroke, diabetes, and so on, but it does next to nothing for weight loss.

That's another weight-loss "dirty little secret." Magazines and books tout walking as the weight-loss solution when, quite frankly, it's not. Do *you* know anyone who has successfully kept a significant amount of weight off when his or her only form of exercise was walking? I've been in this business for more than twenty years, and I don't.

Worse yet are the books that tout cardio as the answer. You cut, cut, cut (calories, that is) and up, up, up your level of cardio. But then you are destined to gain it all back, and then some. Remember, that's exactly what I did when I struggled and repeatedly lost and gained weight. Why did I fail? I killed my *REVVED* opportunity, and I did this damage in my late teens and early twenties. Can you even imagine the damage you are doing if you are in your thirties, forties, fifties, and beyond?

I will give you the lowdown in chapter 7, but suffice it to say that classic cardio performed over a long period actually chews up your precious calorie-burning muscle for fuel. Did you ever wonder why all the people on the cardio machines at the gym seem to constantly battle getting fatter, especially in the midsection? I see that all the time. Yep, not exercising at all is bad, but long-term cardio is even worse when it comes to gaining fat and weight, because it burns up your precious long, lean, calorie-burning, sexy muscle. Yes, the long-term cardio has numerous health benefits, such as reducing the risk of heart disease and cancer, but it's a total bust when it comes to weight and fat loss. As hard as this is to believe, at least now you know why your past attempts didn't achieve your ultimate result: a leaner, lighter you.

The research is clear. Lose weight without strength training and generally the weight lost will be 50 percent fat—that's good—and 50 percent muscle—that's really, really bad, especially when you learn that, with age, we are all losing muscle. It starts as early as our twenties. And women, if you are anywhere near menopause (which, FYI, is happening earlier and earlier these days), the rate at which you lose muscle starts to double. You are wondering, "What's happening to me? My old diet tricks don't work. My waist is thickening. My body has taken on a life of its own." That's happening because you are in metabolic free fall. Don't despair. I will help you reverse that trend, and it is possible that you can achieve the best shape of your life in your forties, fifties, and older.

Guys, don't think the concept of "male menopause" is fiction. Our hormones change (mostly decreasing) as we age, we lose human growth hormone and testosterone, and a whole host of other chemical changes occur, *not* for the better. Although male menopause is not as tested or understood as female menopause, both women *and* men need *REVVED* behaviors to manage the aging process, especially during those tricky years in the late forties and fifties.

Have you noticed what happens to people later in life? The average person loses 3 pounds of muscle—a year—after the age of seventy. That could easily be the difference between an independent and dependent lifestyle going forward. We all pay attention to socking away funds for our retirement, but are you actively thinking about building muscle mass as you age? If you truly love and care about those around you who are at or approaching that age, please hand them a copy of this book; it's life-altering.

Cleanses

***REVVED* Fiction**	"A cleanse burns fat." That's totally false. Just about all a cleanse does is burn your precious calorie-burning muscle and deplete you of your essential "fat-burning" water.
***REVVED* Fact**	Classic diets kill your *REVVED* goals, but cleanses obliterate it, annihilate it, and make weight gain more efficient than ever before.

Water is considered "fat burning" because of the relationship between the kidneys and the liver:

> The kidneys' primary function is to process waste products. In a well-hydrated body, the kidneys are efficiently able to perform all that needs to be done. Mission accomplished.

> The liver's primary function is to take stored fat and turn it into energy for your body to use. We like that function a lot and want it to be *REVVED* up at all times.

Unfortunately, when the body is dehydrated, the kidneys say "Help" or "Mission *can't* be accomplished" to the liver, and the liver steps in to help process waste products, its secondary function. Therefore, the liver's primary function, basically orchestrating stored fat to be burned for fuel, is diminished. When you ask too much of the liver, it divides its efforts. That "division of responsibility" put the brakes on fat burning. Don't tell your liver to do that by going on a cleanse, which is going to intentionally rid your body of water.

Let's be honest, a cleanse *craze* has swept the country these past few years. I bet you, a very close family member, coworker, or friend has done one. I can't tell you how many people—clients, nonclients, men, women, young, old, whatever—come to me postcleanse, devastated, depressed, and heavier and fatter than ever before. They are crushed and terribly confused and say flat out, "What happened?" as they point to their ever expanding body.

The math is simple. They go on a total liquid cleanse, which is generally devoid of any protein or solid food, and they shed weight fast, but the vast majority of what they lose is muscle and water. Then, when they go back to precleanse eating, the weight comes back, and it's *all* fat. Plus, hormonally, they have compromised their body. It's going to take time, effort, and a smart strategy to get the body hormonally back in balance.

In addition, the cleanse directions probably said to eliminate all exercise. I've seen it in black and white, and I'm shocked. They tell you that when you have absolutely *no* energy to exercise, or do much of anything else for that matter. Therefore, being told "Don't exercise" gives you the license to "just skip it." The cleanse manufacturer knows the scale will go down that much more as you deplete your body of muscle. But you are thrilled with what you see when you step on the scale, so you are "all in" and raring to go cleanse and then . . . gain weight . . . again.

Your *REVVED* opportunity is gone, but the cleanse companies continue to make more money as you feel the need to then cleanse again—to see that number again for a fleeting moment—and ruin your metabolism that much more. Both your metabolism and your body's composition are shot. Depressing, if you ask me.

The yo-yo effect is brutal on the body. You are sending the body mixed signals. It's like a bad relationship that you keep going back to:

I love you, but I think we should see other people.

I love you, but maybe it's best if we *not* move in together.

I love you, but I want a R-E-A-L-L-Y long engagement.

Would you encourage any of your friends to give this relationship the go-ahead? That's what you are doing every time you cleanse and expect a lasting outcome.

You really think the weight is going to *stay* off this time? Come on.

The physicians my firm in Chicago and New York works closely with report the same experience. Women *and* men are coming into their offices in droves with weight gain, hormonal imbalances, deep frustration, and depression, *all* as a result of their cleanse addiction.

I do believe it's an addiction. First, it's an addiction to a number on the scale, even though it's only attained for about 24 hours. How many of you know your "postcleanse" number? It's almost as memorable as your wedding-day weight.

Second, I believe cleansing is an addiction to the quick fix. "Oh, I've got a 'red carpet' or high school reunion (or some other event) in two weeks. Let's cleanse." Then insanity once again rears its ugly head as you really *do* expect the weight to stay off this time. No, no, no, that's not going to happen—because it can't.

Finally, it's an addiction to the power. You attend a luncheon, sit down with your bottle of juice, and beam as you tell your friends, "I'm on day three of my cleanse," which means, "Look at me! I'm taking control of my body." It's empowering but, at the same time, so very, very wrong.

Although I loathe (isn't it clear?) cleanses, I do like men and women who "own up" to their weight-loss goals. Chapter 3 of my first book, *The Business Plan for the Body,* is called "Going Public." In that chapter, I tell my readers to let everyone—friends, family members, and coworkers—know that their goal was permanent weight loss. I love it when people confidently say, with a smile, "I'm on the *REVVED* weight-loss plan." Trust me, all eyes will be on you as your friends, family members, and co-workers *should* be interested to hear what you are doing. You *should* be honest about your desire, your need, your hope, to live a healthier, leaner life. If those around you don't like it, well, read on.

Why did I keep italicizing *should*? I did because there is also a second issue in play when it comes to your friends and that has to do with what is coined "network contagion," which is a trio of mechanisms involved with friend selection that include

- social influence

- social environment

- social selection

Researchers debate which of the three factors affects weight more than the others, but one in particular, Charles F. Manski, from the University of Wisconsin at Madison, cites the "reflection problem" and believes all three issues truly mirror each other. I agree with him.[2]

In my over two decades in the weight-loss industry I have found that the number-one factor that affects your body weight are the people you hang around with most frequently. I agree that people often choose friends of a similar size, who like to hang around similar environments and that the behavior in those environments is similar. Think for a moment of your own friends. Are they similar in size to you? Do they eat, drink, sleep, and exercise like you? Do you talk about similar desires and are some of those desires weight loss, enhanced body composition, *REVVED*-up energy levels, and a longer, healthier life? You tell me.

You may be surprised by what you realize when thinking about the answers to these questions. Did you pick certain friends because you possess the same habits? It can be both a plus and a minus. I know so many people who met their future spouse at places like a health club (mutual interest in working out) or at church (mutual interest in faith). I also know couples who met because they both went outside during a party to smoke. The issue that you have to wrestle with is, are your friends going to encourage you to adopt the *REVVED* behaviors or are you going to get resistance? Do your own analysis as you go, but don't be surprised if you get the "Are you just going to eat protein and vegetables—again?" comments from those who don't like your desire for improvement. Similarly, you will get the people, some of whom you have only met once or twice, who come up to you and say, "You inspire me. Please tell me what you have going differently, because you just look great and seem happier." I say be bold. Be proud, but be prepared. Wear your weight-loss plan, and its success, with pride and inspire others. Be an active part of this *REVO*lution!

What about a juice cleanse? You might as well just fill a bowl with sugar and dive in, because that's pretty much what you are getting, as there are practically *no* nutrients and vitamins in most store-bought juice cleanses.

So what about a juice cleanse you do at home, where you take a bunch of fruit and veggies and toss them in a juicer? Once again, I have issues:

1. **Where's the protein?** Some vegetables contain a little protein, but not nearly enough. To give you an idea, 1 cup of chopped broccoli contains about 2½ grams of protein. It will take 36 cups of broccoli for women and 48 for men to get you to an acceptable level of approximately 90 ounces a day for women and 120 ounces for men. That's your *REVVED* protein requirement, and it's all done for you in the *REVVED* Eating Plan.

    The issue of protein consumption is critical, because low intake will cause the body to shed muscle at an even faster rate. I've established that you lose 50 percent muscle and 50 percent fat on most traditional diets that do not include strength training. But the amount of muscle loss can be slightly minimized by increasing the amount of protein intake on a diet. Eating more protein while on a calorie-restricted diet can spare *some* of the muscle loss, but you will still lose muscle if you neglect your strength training.

2. **Your blood sugar will spike, followed by a blood sugar "crash."** Juice packs a ferocious, quick, empty punch, and you will learn what happens after that in the next chapter.

3. **Juice and other liquid calories don't trigger satiety mechanisms.** I'm going to give you the whole story on that in chapter 5.

We all see celebrities go up and down in weight with astonishing speed. I believe weight loss keeps a lot of magazines in business. Really, another cover story on celebrity X's weight gain and then, three months later, weight loss? Trust me, they are *all* cleansing or doing something just as drastic. I know from close friends who are therapists that the depression that comes when the weight piles back on with a vengeance postcleanse is catastrophic. Just know that depression is partly because of the embarrassment and partly because of the hormonal imbalance that resulted. It's a bad one-two punch in every way. Physicians can see the imbalance from the results of certain blood tests. As I've said, hormones do play a big role in successful weight loss. Therefore, shocking your body with a cleanse followed by a big weight gain gives your body the wrong signal and affects a number of hormones, including insulin, leptin, ghrelin, and especially the feel-good hormone serotonin. If you give your body mixed signals, it's simply confused, and part of that confusion leads to hormonal imbalance.

Please don't ever diet without *REVVED* behaviors. And never, ever cleanse.

The REVVED Eating Rules

4

Before I give you the detailed 28-day *REVVED* Eating Plan (chapter 6), I want to share the eating rules, which include what has led to the tremendous success of my clients but also my interpretation of research.

"The Hunger Games"

In the blockbuster books and movie entitled *The Hunger Games*, twenty-four young men and woman are randomly selected to participate in a live televised "fight to the death" event. Only one will be crowned the winner, and the rest will lose in a big way—they'll die! The title of this series spoke volumes to me, as I strongly believe our current obesity and overweight epidemic proves that we are losing the "hunger games."

***REVVED* Fiction**   "Skipping meals is a smart weight-loss strategy."

***REVVED* Fact**   You can control hunger.

Hunger and blood sugar go hand in hand. When you are hungry, you are experiencing a drop in blood sugar. There is only one time during the day you should ever be hungry: first thing in the morning. Look at the fact that you have been on an 8 to 10 hour fast, depending on when you ate dinner and when you got up. Why do you think we call it break*fast*? I know I get up ravenous and can't wait to hit the kitchen for one of my biggest meals of the day. (Did you catch that? Yes, one of my *biggest* meals of the day.) After that time, I never allow myself to feel hunger again until the following morning. And no, this doesn't mean I snack every 2 hours to ward off hunger. Rather, I eat three balanced meals and one postexercise snack each day. Balanced meals consist of lean proteins, healthy fats, portioned carbohydrates, and lots of satiating colorful vegetables. I'll go over the *REVVED* balanced meal plan later in this chapter.

REVVED Fiction   "If you don't eat fat, you won't get fat."

REVVED Fact   Eating the right fats keeps you from feeling hungry.

Do you remember the no- and low-fat craze that started in the late 1980s? Some supposed experts said, "If you don't eat fat, you won't get fat," and the whole "fat-free" phenomenon was launched. It was quite possibly some of the worse advice ever given, as this led many people (including me) to eat predominately fat-free foods. What a disaster.

British researchers found that when a product is labeled "fat-free," consumers eat approximately 50 percent more of it.[1] Oh, not good.

> I totally agree with the British researchers, because I know I ate more fat-free products and witnessed my clients doing the same. Although this was before I learned that fat-free products (note, these are manufactured products and not fruits and vegetables, which are naturally fat-free) are one of the worst possible choices you can make, but I was petrified to eat fat and instructed my clients to avoid it as much as possible. I would go so far as to call myself "fat-phobic." Remember, it's now known that fat is good, as it triggers satiety and keeps you feeling full longer. Fat is also essential for optimal vitamin storage. We want those anti-aging, disease-reducing vitamins running rampant in our bodies, and fat helps that happen.

Why was this belief and the behavior that resulted such a disaster? Fat-free sweet carbohydrates (such as cookies, cakes, muffins, etc.) and many of the classic processed carbs (such as white bread, bagels, rice, pasta, pretzels, etc.) along with the big killers soda and juice are what I refer to as quick, empty foods.

When you get up in the morning and eat breakfast, that's good. But if that breakfast is a white bagel, that's bad. The white processed carb is going to very quickly leave your stomach and become glucose (blood sugar). Carbohydrates, especially processed carbs, turn *very* quickly to glucose. Protein and fats must be broken down and rebuilt, meaning they take longer to digest, and you will soon learn why a slower, longer transition to glucose is ideal for your *REVVED*. Glucose can be either used for fuel (once again, that's good) or stored in your liver and muscle as fat (that's bad). All food may ultimately turn into glucose, depending on the needs of the body. The issue is that simple carbs cause a rapid increase in your blood glucose level, which signals insulin to store glucose (energy) as quickly as possible. Our bodies have a limited capacity to store glucose as glycogen, so when we consume too many carbs, they get stored as fat. It's important to note that the more physically fit our bodies are, the more glycogen our muscles and liver can store. That is why it is essential to incorporate both a healthy diet and strength training to boost metabolism. My *REVVED* Exercise Plan will enable your muscles to store more glycogen, which means that after you eat a balanced meal, the glucose will be sent to your muscles and will not be stored as fat.

So, the white bagel being quickly turned into glucose results in your having a big sugar party going on in your bloodstream. High blood sugar is what diabetics have to manage, and all of us know it's serious. I roll my eyes when someone tells me they have a "little" sugar problem. It's not going to stay "little" for long, unless you do something about it.

Now that you have started the "sugar party," that very smart body of yours springs into action. It says, "Wow, there is quite a sugar *bash* going on in here. I need to shut it down," and it instructs the pancreas to produce insulin. Think of insulin as the drawbridge that enables the glucose to enter your cells. Serious diabetics, both type 1 and type 2, inject insulin or take medication to enable the sugar to leave the bloodstream. When you accost the body with a big sugar party by eating processed carbs, the body responds by sending out a big dose of insulin to clear it out, and after that you are left with a drop in blood sugar, a crash in energy, and *hunger*.

You just lost the game.

There are three ways to win this hunger game:

1. **Increase fiber intake.** Fiber is found in many foods, such as fruits, vegetables, legumes, sprouted 100 percent whole-grain carbohydrates (such as oatmeal or quinoa), and nuts, to name a few. Visualize fiber turning your stomach into an hourglass, so that you get a slow drip of food turning into glucose followed by a slow drip of insulin. Translation: consistent blood-sugar and energy levels, and hunger eradicated. You are on your way to winning the game.

2. **Eat well-balanced meals.** When you see the *REVVED* Eating Plan in chapter 6, you will notice that all three meals each day, with only the lunch being slightly lower in calories, are substantial. The 150-calorie fat-free yogurt is no longer breakfast. That sad turkey sandwich with mayo on white bread with a bag of chips is no longer lunch. You aren't going to just "wing it" when it comes to dinner and think you are going to make a smart selection when you are tired, hungry, and stressed out from the day. Those are past behaviors. Now, with just a little extra thought and planning, you will navigate hunger simply because you made smarter, balanced, whole-food meal choices. Balanced meals go way beyond staying within a narrow calorie range. *REVVED* meals consist of a balanced number of carbohydrates, protein, and fat. Later in this chapter I will provide a breakdown of how to balance these macronutrients to boost your metabolism.

3. **Increase protein.** There is so much to say about protein that I want to save that discussion for later. Just know that it's a big *REVVED* contributor. Let me just say that eating a high-protein breakfast in comparison to a high-carbohydrate breakfast is much more effective in reducing the hunger hormone, ghrelin, after the meal, as a study at TNO Quality of Life, Zeist, the Netherlands, proved.[2] Suffice it to say that keeping ghrelin levels low stimulates a *REVVED* body:

Hunger Down = *REVVED* Up

*REV*erse Your Caloric Intake

In the *REVVED* Eating Plan, you are going to eat three balanced meals and one snack. For the 1,200-Calorie Meal Plan, breakfast and dinner are approximately 400 calories each, lunch is approximately 300 calories, and the snack is 100 calories. For the 1,600-calorie meal plan, breakfast and dinner are approximately 500 calories each, lunch is approximately 400 calories, and the snack is 200 calories. You will consume the majority of your calories before 3:00 P.M., which you will soon learn is advisable for accelerated weight loss.

I allowed the larger dinner simply to up the chances that you will actually comply with the plan. As I said earlier, if the research absolutely proves that dinner should be small for weight loss, will people outside of a laboratory setting really sit at a restaurant with a dinner salad and 3 ounces of grilled chicken? I don't think so. That's why I went with the smart solution and allowed you to eat a slightly larger dinner. Also, by eating a balanced, larger dinner, you will feel satiated until you wake up the next morning. No more midnight snacks or after-dinner eating, because you now know they have disastrous consequences for your HGH, human growth hormone, which is so essential to your *REVVED* metabolism. To me, that just makes sense.

Eat the Majority of Your Calories *Early*

A study by Marta Garaulet and Frank Scheer, director of the medical chronobiology program at Brigham and Women's Hospital in Boston, followed 420 people in Spain for a twenty-week experiment. All participants were on a restricted-calorie diet, but those who ate their biggest meals before 3:00 P.M. lost 5 *more* pounds than those who ate later. The early eaters lost 22 pounds, while the later eaters lost only 17 when on the exact same eating plan. They consumed exactly the same calories; the only variable was when the food was eaten. That's pretty compelling.[3]

Researchers aren't completely sure why this occurred, but they believe one issue may be the fact that consuming more of your calories earlier in the day rather than later (which is atypical American behavior) may over time enhance insulin functionality. The takeaway message is that

- spacing out balanced meals every 4 to 5 hours (which is your *REVVED* strategy and what the participants did in the study) may be a more effective way to achieve optimal body weight, compared to "saving" calories for later in the day; and

- consuming the majority of your calories before 3:00 P.M. may prevent the habitual snacking that occurs by those who consume the majority of their calories after 3:00 P.M. That habitual snacking is going to call upon insulin over and over again, and our goal is to minimize calling upon it, as it is a storage hormone.

A study reported in *Obesity* found the same results in rats. When eating the same high-fat diet,

rats that ate before going to bed gained 48 percent more body fat, but

rats that ate earlier *only* gained 20 percent more body fat.[4]

Once again, same calorie diet, significant difference in weight gained. The only variable: timing. Compelling.

REVerse Your Belief System

If you believe in saving your calories for later in the day, I want you to turn your current belief system around. You probably behave something like I did, before I saw the light (and lost a lot of weight).

Jim Karas's Old Belief System and Behavior

I would skip or scrimp on breakfast. I was so proud of myself when I would rush to work or to my workout first thing (100 percent cardio, 100 percent of the time, as I so *believed* it would work) after eating *nothing* or maybe, just maybe, an orange. Translation: 100 calories. Done!

At lunch, it was a little salad with barely any dressing or maybe a fat-free yogurt and another piece of fruit. Translation: 200 calories. "Look at me, look at me, I'm so proud of myself for starving" was what I thought. I wore it like a "Badge of Smart."

Then, around 3:00 P.M. extreme hunger pangs would hit. I would go for a 250-calorie bag of pretzels ("Hey, they're fat-free!") and a 250-calorie bag of fat-free microwave popcorn. Translation: 500 calories. "But I've been so *good* today," I thought. "I'm only at 800 calories (yes, I counted every one) and haven't eaten any fat (another flawed behavior)."

I got home at 6:00 P.M., totally starving (I was thinking about food all the way home, and you can only imagine how my blood sugar was plummeting), and the evening cabal began. I would throw my coat on a chair and immediately dig into some cheese and crackers (actually, a lot of cheese and crackers—it had to be 500 calories, maybe more), eaten while standing at the kitchen counter. Okay, now I was at 1,300 calories. Sometimes I popped the cork off a bottle of wine, especially when I was with friends, so let's add another 300 calories for two nice 6-ounce glasses of wine at 150 each. I'm at 1,600 calories, and that's not so bad, but I haven't had dinner—yet.

I was knee-deep in the "danger zone," because I was still really hungry and about to "have at" some serious caloric intake. I settled into dinner, which consisted of grilled chicken and rice that I had bought at a healthy prepared-food section, which, truthfully, was loaded with oil, and a container of green beans, super-packed with good stuff but, like the rice and chicken, with a lot of added fat. I'd say I ate a good 800 calories for dinner. You know, not so bad when I was only now at 2,400 calories for the day.

And I had eaten pretty good stuff—some fruit, a yogurt, some fat-free carbs, cheese, crackers, grilled chicken, rice, and veggies. Come on, was that so bad? Plus, remember from chapter 1, I can eat close to 2,651 (my AMR), so that's good—"I've been good"—but I wasn't done.

Nope, it was ice cream and cookie time. I bought the reduced or fat-free ice cream or frozen yogurt, but I was able to polish off the entire small container, which was four servings at 150 calories a serving. That added 600 calories to my 2,400. I was now hitting 3,000 calories. But wait, I thought, I did work out that morning (1 hour of steady-state cardio, remember?) after my one orange, so why couldn't I have four 100-calorie fat-free cookies? And I was still a little hungry . . .

I now understand why I was still hungry. Look at all those simple carbs in my day, the fat-free pretzels and popcorn, the crackers, the rice, the ice cream and cookies, and the fact that I created an environment where insulin must have been pumping all day and into the night. And you wonder why I was still hungry after all the food at night? It's because I didn't trigger satiety, as I ate virtually nothing for breakfast and lunch and had fat only in my cheese and chicken and some added oil on my rice and beans. Couple that with the fact that I was still flooded, right before going to bed, with insulin, which was only making me even hungrier and telling—no, demanding—that my body store fat (and shut down the production of human growth hormone, which I already explained).

As my head hit the pillow after I had eaten 3,400 calories, 75 percent of which I consumed *after* 6:00 P.M., I wondered, "Why won't my weight go down? I starved myself most of the day. Is it my genes?"

It wouldn't go down because I didn't tell it to go down. My beliefs and behaviors were so distorted that I kept thinking, "There must be some other problem, as I'm really a smart eater."

I was smart—not!—and let's keep in mind, this was a weekday and a workday. What are most of your weekdays like in comparison to your weekends, when you are hanging around the house during the day and going out at night?

My beliefs and behaviors kept me overweight and frustrated.

Milton Stokes, chief dietitian for St. Barnabas Hospital in New York City, says, "Breakfast skippers replace calories during the day with mindless nibbling, bingeing at lunch and dinner. They set themselves up for failure."[5] Again, that was me.

Then I saw the light. Now you will too. I was starving myself, so the body did what I told it to: It demanded more food later in the day, knowing that an unwanted "fast" was going to happen that night and again the next day.

And even *more* research agrees. Elisabetta Politi, nutrition manager for the Duke Diet and Fitness Center at Duke University Medical School, says, "Eating early also jump-starts your metabolism. When you don't eat breakfast, you're actually fasting for 15 to 20 hours, so you're not producing the enzymes needed to metabolize fat to lose weight."[6]

"Not producing the enzymes needed to metabolize fat to lose weight." Isn't that what your *REVVED* machine is all about?

Start *REV*ing your day with a big *balanced* breakfast. Again, this is the total opposite of what I did for years when I was overweight. When I go out to breakfast with people (which I love to do), they are shocked by what I order:

3 poached eggs = 270 calories

3 pieces of chicken sausage = 150 calories

2 cups or 2 pieces of fruit = 200 calories

1 piece of Ezekiel or other sprouted-grain toast, and if they don't have that, classic whole-wheat or whole-grain toast = 100 calories

Lots and lots of green tea, either hot or cold = 0 calories

That's a 720-calorie breakfast, and I can eat 2,651 calories a day to maintain my weight. Aside from the 720 calories, this meal has a balanced portion of carbohydrates (from the fruit and toast) and a healthy amount of protein and fat (from the eggs and sausage) to promote satiety, muscle repair, and balanced hormones. It's important to note that 2,651 calories per day for me is weight maintenance. If I wanted to lose weight, I would have to create a caloric deficit.

Please note that 720 calories also represents about 27 percent of my daily caloric intake. By 3:00, I will have consumed between 65 and 75 percent of my daily caloric intake, give or take, so that gives me a lot to fill up on during the day.

Timing of Meals = *REVVED* Behavior

The timing of meals is getting more and more attention. When I say timing, I mean eating at the same time of day, every day, for approximately the same amount of time. The Hebrew University of Jerusalem conducted a case study on four different groups of mice that all ate the same number of calories. The only difference was the fat content of their food and their eating schedule.

Carbohydrates

The carbohydrates that you will be consuming on the *REVVED* plan will be predominately from fruits, vegetables, legumes, nuts, seeds, and some sprouted 100 percent whole-wheat or whole-grain sources. You aren't going to consume white, processed, refined carbs during these first, critical 28 *REV*olutionary days, and I hope you will continue to shun them in your diet going forward.

Why should you opt for sprouted grains? Sprouted grains are less processed than the majority of the "whole-grain" products you see on the shelves. Many whole-grain products go through a slew of manufacturing procedures that mitigate their nutritional benefits. Sprouted grains, on the other hand, are still intact at the time of consumption. Furthermore, most sprouted breads are lower on the glycemic index than 100 percent whole-wheat products, which means that you won't experience a dramatic spike in blood glucose levels. Finally, sprouted grains contain less phytic acid than nonsprouted grains. Phytic acid binds to, and thus makes unabsorbable, minerals such as iron, calcium, zinc, and magnesium—all essential nutrients to support a healthy immune system and metabolism.

I also want to dispel another myth: that fruit prevents weight loss and should be prohibited on a diet plan. I love fruit. My clients and followers enjoy fruit. No one thinks fruit is off limits who understands the following:

- Fruit has fiber, which is essential to maintaining consistent blood-sugar levels and managing hunger. Foods containing fiber also generally require us to chew longer, which helps trigger satiety. Fiber also keeps you regular, helps lower cholesterol, and reduces the risk of heart disease, some cancers, and stoke.

- Fruit contains vitamins and minerals essential to a *REVVED* metabolism and to a disease-free, anti-inflammatory, energized mind and body.

- Fruit contains water, which we talked about in chapter 3. You will learn in chapter 5 that you can drink *and* eat water (hint: fruits and vegetables are packed with water).

Of course, you can consume too much of a good thing. Fruit is a simple sugar (mostly fructose), and if you consume copious amounts all day long, your body releases insulin, which will ultimately prevent fat loss. On the *REVVED* Eating Plan, I've incorporated about two servings of fruit per day. This is enough to provide an ample number of antioxidants and enough sweetness to satisfy a sweet tooth.

Here are some basic rules when consuming fruit:

1. **Choose whole fruits, such as apples and berries.** Avoid all juice; juice is really no different from soda (although it may contain a few antioxidants— more on that in chapter 5) with regard to its ability to jack up blood-glucose levels.

2. **Avoid dried fruit, as it is concentrated sugar.** Think of a handful of raisins (about 15). Pretty easy to overindulge with raisins. However, 15 grapes (about 1 cup) would be a much more filling portion.

3. **Never consume fruit on its own.** Always pair it with a protein or fat to help minimize a spike in blood sugar. For example, enjoy an apple with some cheese or nut butter.

4. **Go green!** When choosing which type of fruit to eat, you might reach for green apples, as the combination of tart and sweet has been shown to trigger satiety that much more.

Fat

Fat gets a bad rap. It shouldn't. I talked earlier about the disaster that ensued following the whole "fat-free" phenomenon. Don't ever consume a fat-free product unless it is a whole food that occurs naturally that way. You may even be surprised to see foods that contain saturated fat are a part of the *REVVED* Eating Plan. Those *approved* foods that do contain saturated fat include meat, butter, cage-free eggs, and coconut oil, to name a few. The fat that you should avoid comes from processed foods, where trans fat is used, hydrogenated fat (used in foods such as margarine), and pressed seed oils, such as soybean and canola oil.

Essential fatty acids are just that, essential to a *REVVED* body. Fatty acids are straight-chain molecules formed from the elements carbon, hydrogen, and oxygen. The bonds between the elements determine the length of the chain and type of fat. There are three types of chains: short, medium, and long.

Short-chain fatty acids contain fewer than six carbons and are found in dairy products from grass-fed cows. These short-chain fatty acids, among them butyric and caproic acids, are beneficial for maintaining a healthy digestive tract.

Medium-chain fatty acids contain between six and twelve carbons and are found in coconut and palm oil. Both oils contain caprylic, capric, and lauric acids. Interestingly, in a case study when olive oil was replaced with one of these two oils, participants in the study actually lost *more* weight.[10] I wonder if olive oil just has a bigger lobby in Washington or a better public-relations firm, because as all we hear about is "olive oil, olive oil, olive oil," when some of the other oils are truly more beneficial to the body, especially where weight loss is concerned.

A study published in the *American Journal of Clinical Nutrition* reported that "medium-chain fatty acids were three times more effective at raising the metabolism than long-chain fatty acids." Another study from the same journal showed that "eating medium-chain fatty acids increases metabolism and also helps burn off stored fat."[11]

Sounds very *REVVED* to me.

But wait! Coconut oil also

1. slows digestion, so that you feel full longer;

2. prevents blood-sugar fluctuations; and

3. destroys candida, which is yeast overgrowth in the body. A regular amount of yeast is beneficial, but when it becomes excessive, there are many adverse consequences, one of which is increased cravings for sugar, bread, pasta, and other carbohydrates, *plus* alcohol. We know we want to minimize cravings for these foods, so a *REVVED* behavior would be to add coconut oil to your meals.[12]

Long-chain fatty acids contain more than twelve carbons and are found in meat, fish, cocoa, nuts, seeds, and vegetable oils. These foods contain palmitic, oleic, and stearic acids.

Avoid long-chain fatty acids found in processed food and factory-farmed meats. Also avoid what are termed highly refined vegetable oils, such as safflower, sunflower, cottonseed, and soy. These oils become oxidized when subjected to heat, oxygen, and moisture, which occurs in cooking and processing. When oxidized, they frequently become free radicals, which attack cell membranes, red blood cells, protein, lipids, and DNA. This terrible inflammatory damage accelerates aging and chronic illness, such as heart disease, diabetes, arthritis, and cancer.[13]

Long-chain omega-3 fatty acids trigger or help you to achieve satiety. In one research study with overweight or obese individuals on a calorie-restricted diet, those who ate more long-chain omega-3 fatty acids (greater than 1,300 milligrams) reported feeling more satisfied following a similar meal that contained less than 260 milligrams.[14] Once again, if a food helps trigger satiety and doesn't include any seriously detrimental elements, then I feel it should be included in the *REVVED* Eating Plan.

Conjugated linoleic acid (CLA) is found in butter made from the cream of grass-fed cows. You will see it in the *REVVED* Eating Plan. Conjugated linoleic acid is a trans fat, but it is actually a good, naturally occurring one. It has also been associated with accelerated fat loss, and the researchers agree. I've been "antibutter" for years, but the benefits of grass-fed butter for fat loss, satiety, and taste can no longer be ignored. So enjoy your butter—odds are, if you are like me, your taste buds will pop when it's added to some of your meals.

Short- and medium-chain fatty acids are quickly absorbed, as they are easy to digest. A classic example of a short-chain fatty acid is butter, while medium-chain fatty acids include butter (as it possesses both short- and medium-chain fatty acids), milk, yogurt, cheese, coconut and palm-kernel oils, to name a few. They don't require a lot of work. Long-chain fatty acids require enzymes provided by the liver, so they do take longer to digest.

Fish oil contains the omega-3 fatty acids EPA (eicosapentaenoic acid) and DHA (docosahexaenoic acid). DHA is found in algae and fish; however, EPA is only found in fish. Researchers from the University of Western Ontario found that fish oil may have the power to dramatically boost your metabolism by about 400 calories per day.[15] That's a big number. They found that fish oil increases levels of fat-burning enzymes and decreases levels of fat-storage enzymes in your body. Although I have included fish in your *REVVED* Eating Plan and you will derive fish-oil benefits from it, my recommendation would be to also supplement. As always, consult with your doctor before adding any type of supplement. Choose capsules containing a total of at least 300 milligrams of EPA and DHA for the optimal metabolic boost, and you may also want to find a high-quality fish oil that has been purified to eliminate mercury.[16]

Protein

Protein is critically important to your *REVVED* machine because it:

1. **Increases satiety.** Think of satiety as a derivation of the word "satisfied"; increasing satiety directly results in a feeling of fullness and *less hunger*. There have been numerous studies that have shown this to be true, but a study on sixty-five overweight and obese individuals in 1999 illustrates my point. The instructions were simple: One group was to consume 25 percent of their daily caloric intake in protein (the HP group, for "high protein"), while the second group was instructed to consume only 12 percent of their calories in protein (the NP, or "normal protein," group).

   At the end of the six-month study, the results were dramatically different: The HP group lost an average of 19.6 pounds. The NP group lost only 11.2 pounds. Remember, the participants were not put on a specific calorie-restricted diet. They were only given protein guidelines. The researchers theorized that the high protein content helped to trigger satiety mechanisms, therefore reducing the total daily caloric intake and creating more of a caloric deficit.[17]

2. **Possesses a high thermic effect, which is the energy used to digest, absorb, and then distribute nutrients.** Protein's thermic effect may be as high at 35 percent, which means that when you consume 100 calories of protein, 35 of the calories will be used for this thermic effect. That leaves your body with only 65 remaining calories. And all the time that protein spends in digestion, absorption, and distribution keeps you feeling full. If protein is going to be stored as body fat, it may take another 50 percent of those remaining 65 calories to facilitate that process, leaving your body with a little over 30 calories to store. Sounds good to me.

3. **Preserves muscle.** As I told you in chapter 1, when you are on a reduced-calorie diet, without strength training you are going to lose muscle. You should now know that this is a fact. As I previously said, by increasing protein intake, you reduce some of the loss of muscle, but by no means all. But we are adding strength training, as it's essential to a *REVVED* outcome. No risk of muscle loss here, though we do need the increased protein, which is made up of amino acids, since it provides the building blocks of our precious calorie-burning muscle.[18]

Lean red meat, skinless chicken and turkey, fish, and seafood are well-known, good sources of protein, but here is a list of some of my favorites that I will add to your *REVVED* meals:

1. **Eggs.** I consider eggs a superfood. A study published in the *American Journal of Clinical Nutrition* asked participants to eat one of two breakfasts, both with the same number of calories: 3 scrambled eggs and 1½ pieces of toast *or* 1 plain bagel, ½ tablespoon of low-fat cream cheese, and 6 ounces of low-fat yogurt. In comparison to those who ate the bagel breakfast, the egg-breakfast participants reduced their consumption, 3 hours later, at a lunch buffet (unlimited options and refills) by 112 calories; consumed approximately 400 fewer calories over the next 24 hours, which equaled a reduction of 18 percent of their daily calories; and produced lower levels of ghrelin, the hunger-inducing hormone, with regard to sleep.[19] This study supported previous research that found egg eaters lost 65 percent more weight and were far more energetic—*REVVED* up—than those who ate a bagel breakfast. That study also compared meals of the exact same calories.[20]

   And don't skip the yolk, as it contains half the protein of the egg and all the fat. I totally believe that the combination of the protein and fat that is in the whole egg provides the one-two punch of satiety. Plus, eggs contain all nine essential amino acids, the true building blocks of muscle.

   Note: If you are at all concerned about the cholesterol in eggs, know that recent research found that eggs contain more protein and less cholesterol than we originally thought.

Eggs are an excellent source of choline. Choline has been found to help play a role in turning off unfavorable genes and improving DNA methylation. So if you are cursed with bad genes, remember to eat the yolk!

REVVED Fiction	"Eating fat-free will keep you from getting fat." "Starving makes you thin." Now add "Eggs are bad for you."
REVVED Fact	All three of these fictions are totally untrue (and this list is going to grow).

2. **Pine nuts.** You may be shocked to know that, of all nuts, pine nuts contain the highest protein content. But, truth be told, pine nuts, though called "nuts," are actually seeds. Pine nuts possess pinolenic acid, a naturally occurring omega-6 fatty acid that stimulates hormones (one is cholecystokinin, which is also in beans) that trigger satiety and provide that *REVVED* fullness. "In one study, women who consumed pinolenic acid reported a decreased desire to eat and also reduced their food intake by 36 percent."[21] You only need to consume one shot glass full as a serving.

3. **Sesame seeds.** Christine Gerbstadt, spokesperson for the Academy of Nutrition and Dietetics, says, "Plant chemicals called lignans in sesame seeds enhance fat burning by increasing liver enzymes that break down fat. Many studies found that protein and essential fatty acids increase the metabolic rate, and sesame seeds are loaded in both."[22] They are also a rich source of fiber. I know. I've been hitting them more and more since reading this research, and I will show you how to add them to your diet in the *REVVED* Eating Plan.

4. **Peanuts.** A study in the *International Journal of Obesity and Related Metabolic Disorders* found that when people consumed 500 calories' worth of peanuts daily for nineteen weeks, their resting metabolism increased by 11 percent. It has also been found that peanuts have a very high thermic effect, so high that they actually burn calories. And once again, peanuts are packed with fiber. Do you see how the whole fiber component consistently reappears when it comes to *REVVED* foods? It's essential to this plan's success. On a side note, peanuts decrease your risk of prostate cancer by up to 40 percent. That a big decrease.[23]

5. **Whey protein.** I drink a shake containing whey protein almost every day. Whey protein triggers satiety hormones, one of which is cholecystokinin, and that is going to make you feel full. I frequently drink a whey protein shake postworkout as my snack. It is the perfect combination of protein, carbohydrates, and fat. I will give you some of my favorite recipes in the next chapter.

Other *REVVED*-Producing Foods

Beans

Only about 30 percent of the calories in beans come from protein; the rest come from carbohydrates. A big plus of beans is that they keep you full, as they are packed with resistant starch. About half the calories from resistant starch consumed cannot actually be absorbed. Therefore, you feel full and get some protein, but it doesn't come at a high calorie cost. Beans possess the hormone cholecystokinin too, which has been shown to act as a natural appetite suppressant. Plus, beans are packed with B vitamins, which keeps metabolism chugging at a high rate, since B vitamins help to metabolize protein, carbohydrates, and fat. Amazingly, they also create a fatty acid that burns fat at a faster pace than would have occurred had the B vitamins not been present. Vanderbilt University showed that vitamin B-6, also known as niacin, when working in tandem with iron increased the production of the amino acid L-carnitine. L-carnitine actually promotes fat burning, which is what we want to accomplish on our *REVVED* Eating Plan.[24] I've included beans in your meal plan, as they appear to me to be a metabolism-boosting, fat-burning phenomenon. Plus, they are a good source of folate, another methylating food that influences our genes! Go beans!

Foods with Vitamin C

Quick, think of a food packed with vitamin C. I bet oranges immediately come to mind. Sure, oranges do have C, but did you know that one yellow pepper contains 341 milligrams of C, nearly three and a half times that of oranges? According to a study in the *Journal of Nutrition,* people with higher vitamin-C levels have lower BMIs and even possess less body fat than those with lower levels. In this study, 118 middle-aged people were tested for vitamin-C levels in their blood. What the researchers found was that those who possessed a BMI lower than 25 (25 is the threshold for being considered overweight and 30 is the threshold for being considered obese) possessed an average vitamin-C level of 54.4μmol/L compared to 37.2μmol/L for those with a BMI greater than 35 (which is 5 points above the obese level of 30).[25] That's a considerable difference.

Why? The researchers point to carnitine, which is involved in what is called "fat oxidation" and involves the breakdown of fatty acids, which can then be used by the body. Carnitine also comes into play with regard to exercise, as it has been shown that *less* carnitine actually reduces the body's ability to call upon fat for energy, which causes a decrease in your body's ability to perform the exercise. It reduces your ability to perform exercise, since the body can't tap into fat for energy. You will learn in chapter 7 that intensity of exercise is key to achieving your *REVVED* goals. Therefore, having a lot of carnitine to activate fat cells for energy is important.

A study published in the *Journal of the American College of Nutrition* in 2005, conducted in the Department of Nutrition at Arizona State University, found that individuals who received an adequate intake of vitamin C oxidized 30 percent more fat during moderate exercise than individuals who were deficient in vitamin C.[26]

You will see many foods rich in vitamin C popping up in the *REVVED* Eating Plan. Here are more foods that pack a vitamin-C punch:

- Red and green bell peppers, in addition to the aforementioned yellow
- Fresh herbs, such as thyme and parsley
- Dark leafy greens
- Broccoli, cauliflower, and Brussels sprouts
- Oranges and clementines
- Strawberries[27]

The Role of Herbs and Spices

A number of herbs and spices provide a good bump in antioxidants in your *REVVED* Eating Plan. Surprisingly, many spices possess more rich, anti-aging, and disease-preventing properties than what you would assume you would derive from fruits, vegetables, tea, and coffee.

Fiber is another benefit. It doesn't seem possible that spices contain fiber, but they do, and I've already explained the magic of fiber and how it slows the stomach's release of food (glucose) and leads to a lower, positive, insulin response, which is what we strive to achieve when following the *REVVED* Eating Plan. Remember, we don't want the sugar party parking in our body. No sugar party is possible when fiber is in the house.

Some of My Favorite REVVED Herbs and Spices

Basil possesses magnesium, iron, calcium, potassium, vitamin C, and high levels of antioxidants. It is beneficial for:

Preventing bacterial growth

Minimizing inflammation (It contains cyclooxygenase, which is found in both aspirin and ibuprofen.)

Heart health (It reduces cholesterol in the bloodstream.)

Reducing stress (It contains phytochemicals shown to reduce cortisol production.)

Chili powder, containing vitamins A and C and flush with phosphorus, potassium, iron, calcium, manganese, selenium, and zinc, can:

Boost metabolism

Relieve achy joints (Capsaicin, found in chili peppers, has an anti-inflammatory effect.)

Reduce the risk of blood clots

Clear mucus from a runny nose or congested lungs

Cilantro, also known as coriander, is rich in magnesium, iron, and phyto-nutrients and has been shown to:

Lower blood sugar, as it is packed with fiber

Help bind to heavy metals in the body (Heavy metals have been found to be rampant in our air, food, and water, and we want them out of our body. By binding with metal in a process called chelation, cilantro helps cleanse our tissues, organs, and even our blood, mitigating the potential damage that could occur from heavy metals.)

Protect against salmonella and reduce nausea

Prevent inflammation, or at least lessen its severity

Reduce hormonal mood swings

Cinnamon possesses manganese, iron, calcium, fiber, and high levels of antioxidants and is beneficial for:

Managing blood sugar by improving insulin response

Minimizing inflammation and pain from arthritis

Reducing LDL, the bad cholesterol

Preventing cancer, or slowing its progression

Losing weight, especially abdominal fat

Cumin is an excellent source of iron, fiber, and protein and is beneficial for:

A healthy immune system, which prevent colds and infections

Digestion and absorption of nutrients

Improving sleep, as it contains vitamin B, a sleep enhancer

Preventing stress-inducing chemicals in the body

Dill, whether fresh or dried, possesses magnesium, iron, fiber, and high levels of antioxidants and is beneficial for:

Protecting you from free radicals and carcinogens

Digestion, as it calms an upset stomach

Reducing tooth and bone loss, since it also contains high levels of calcium

Curing insomnia

Parsley possesses high antioxidant levels of vitamins C and A and the flavonoid luteolin and is beneficial for:

Protecting you from free radicals and carcinogens

Minimizing inflammation and pain from arthritis

Promoting heart heath, as it helps reduce blood pressure and is rich in folic acid, a vital B vitamin

Reducing fluid retention and swelling, or edema

Rosemary contains carnosol, which has been found in studies to be a potent anticancer compound, and is beneficial for:

Aiding digestion, as it calms an upset stomach

Minimizing inflammation, as it inhibits COX–2, an enzyme responsible for inflammation, and excess nitric oxide

Improving mood, and maybe preventing Alzheimer's disease as well as the normal memory loss associated with aging

The *REVVED* Calorie Count for Men and Women

I am going to present an eating plan for women at 1,200 calories a day and men at 1,600 a day in chapter 6. I just want to comment on that for those of you who feel the number of calories in these eating plans is too restrictive and may cause your metabolism to slow down. It won't. I've achieved outstanding success with people eating at these levels with *no* reduction in basal or active metabolic rate. Remember, if you are on a calorie-restricted diet without strength training, you are doomed to diminish your metabolism. But the addition of all *REVVED* behaviors, including strength training, won't allow that to happen, even at these low caloric levels. What will happen is you will lose weight and fat—fast—as you enhance your body's composition.

Liquid REVVED

We have all heard about the benefits of water. Many of you drink it every day, drink it sometimes, or drink it whenever you remember to. However, proper hydration, and not just water, is vital to your *REVVED* metabolism.

Water

Here's what water does for you:

1. **Reduces calorie consumption.** A research study at Virginia Tech found that when participants drank just 2 glasses of water before breakfast, it resulted in 75 fewer calories consumed at their morning meal than when they did not. It seemed that the water acted as a "calorie-free" appetizer, since it was consumed first.[1] Now, I want you to eat a *big* breakfast to trigger the satiety mechanisms I keep addressing. If these 2 glasses of water help you to feel full, then I say go for it, as triggering satiety and the feeling of fullness is a major *REVVED* behavior. In fact, please feel free to drink 2 glasses of water before *any* meal.

   At the University of North Carolina at Chapel Hill, researchers discovered that those who regularly drank water (approximately 52 ounces a day is what they consumed in the study) consume approximately 200 fewer calories a day than those who didn't. If you work the math

   200 calories × 365 days = 73,000 fewer calories a year

2. **Boosts metabolism.** The Virginia Tech team also found that cold water boosts metabolism, as your body has to work harder to raise it to core

temperature. Other research claims that ice water—iced is how I drink most of my water and tea—produces a boost in metabolism. And don't just drink a little. Those who drank 12 glasses of water achieved a higher *REVVED* metabolism than those who only drank 4.[2]

3. **Reduces stress.** I keep saying that you tell your body what you want it to do, both positively and negatively. I've gone on and on about how stress smashes your *REVVED* goals. Guess what? Dehydration is a stress, and a big one, as all your organs, including your brain, require water to function properly. When the body isn't getting what it needs, like the right food, sleep, oxygen, or water, it "stresses out," pumps out cortisol, and puts the brakes on a *REVVED* opportunity.

"Studies have shown that being just half a liter dehydrated can increase your cortisol levels," says Amanda Carlson, director of performance nutrition at Athletes' Performance, a training institute for world-class athletes.[3] Half a liter is approximately 17 ounces. Let's put two pieces of research together. If you drink your 17 ounces before breakfast (as the Virginia Tech research proves you should do), you will eat 75 fewer calories at breakfast. That same 17 ounces may *also* reduce your cortisol level if you are dehydrated. *Fewer* calories (to a point, as I would never want you to starve or eat too little) coupled with *less* cortisol clearly makes starting each day with 17 ounces of water a *REVVED* "go-to" behavior for each day.

I find that the majority of people get up in the morning dehydrated from what they ate and drank the night before. How do I know? I can see the puffiness around their eyes. They look bloated. When you are dehydrated, the very smart body perceives that there is not an adequate amount of water available and holds on to water stored in the body. Similar to what it does when you skip breakfast, or any meal for that matter, the body goes into "defense mode" and stores the remaining water is has available in your outer tissues. That's why feet, hands, eyes, and so on appear swollen.

Dehydrated individuals also experience low energy levels and impaired concentration, as dehydration can cause shrinkage in brain tissue and a decline in cognitive function.[4]

Also don't forget that a symptom of stress is a rapid heart rate and shallow breathing, both of which use up water. So stress plus dehydration makes you even more dehydrated. Your *REVVED* fire is flaming out.

The human body may last weeks without food, but can last very few days without water. Doesn't that hit home the fact that being dehydrated is not going to produce a little cortisol but drop a full-blown cortisol *bomb* on *REV*?

Lemon Water

If you think plain water fuels a *REVVED* metabolism, what about adding lemon to water? For years, I've watched women in France drink hot water with lemon instead of coffee first thing in the morning. I find French women in Paris are predominately lean. I was in Paris for a close friend's fortieth birthday as I was writing this book. Every morning, after my workout, I sat at a desk in my hotel on the Left Bank and watched the parade of stylish, slender Parisian women stroll by as I wrote. I had to wonder, "Is there some magical property to the lemon water or is this just a trend?"

Turns out, there very well might be some magic to the lemon. I am a big fan of Dr. Joseph Mercola, who happens to practice in the western suburbs of Chicago, where I live. He is a huge proponent of the acid/alkaline relationship and maintaining a proper pH balance in your body. Dr. Mercola believes that most Americans are far too acidic as a result of our poor diet, polluted air, contaminated water, and so on, and an overly acidic body is a breeding ground for disease. To counteract the acidic environment, Dr. Mercola recommends certain foods and liquids that put the body in a more alkaline state. One of the simplest additions is lemon.

Funny, but when you think of acidic foods, you probably think of lemons right away. But once ingested in the body, lemon fosters a more alkaline state because of its very low sugar and high alkaline mineral content. Although lemons contain both ascorbic and citric acid, these weak acids are easily metabolized by the body, therefore allowing the mineral content of lemons to alkalize the blood. Visualize the alkaline minerals pushing the ascorbic and citric acid out of the way (since they are metabolized so quickly), so that they can do their alkalizing job. Therefore, I strongly recommend that you add lemon to your water every morning. I do, and I also add it to my tea, whether it is hot or cold. You should do the same.

In addition to placing your body in a more alkaline state, an 8-ounce glass of water (and, to once again build on the research, make that a little over two 8-ounce glasses of water first thing in the morning before breakfast to hit the magic 17 ounces) with a quarter of a lemon squeezed in also:

Supplies vitamins such as C, B complex, calcium, iron, magnesium, and, if you can believe it, more potassium than grapes or apples

Provides pectin fiber, which I earlier stated assists in weight loss by filling you up

Reduces inflammation

Aids digestion and can ease heartburn

Reduces bloating

Promotes healing, which we want to accelerate when you learn all about the benefits of interval-based strength training (Just so you know, faster healing will enable you to increase intensity and that puts *REVVED* on fire—in a very good way.)

Enhances enzyme function, which removes toxins from the body and stimulates your liver[5]

Just to be clear:

- Water powers metabolism.
- Ice water powers it even more.
- Iced lemon water packs the ultimate one–two–three punch for a *REVVED* metabolism.

How Much Water?

How much water do you really need each day? This is a hotly debated topic. The two "standard" recommendations are:

Eight 8-ounce glasses

Divide your body weight by two and that is the number of ounces your body requires

I placed "standard" in quotes because many factors influence your body's water requirement, which include:

1. **Salt or sodium consumption.** Americans are urged to limit sodium to around 2,400 milligrams a day. To put that in perspective,

1 teaspoon (that's teaspoon, not tablespoon) of sodium contains 2,325 milligrams, so right there you are done. If you are fifty-one or older, are African American, or have high blood pressure, diabetes, or chronic kidney disease, you should be taking in no more than 1,000 milligrams a day—and that's *not* a lot of salt. To be honest, salt is essential for fluid balance, muscle strength (it actually influences the contraction and relaxation of your muscles, which is critically important to the *REVVED* Exercise Plan), and nerve function, but the required amount provides for those things. Most Americans are consuming two to three times as much. Along with the dehydration that comes from overconsumption of sodium comes a number of negative reactions in the body.

The list of high-sodium foods is vast, but here are some of the worst:

Fast food

Processed food

Fat-free processed carbohydrates (When they take the fat out, they up the sodium content for flavor and sweetness—I know that the idea of salt making something sweet sounds odd, but it's true.)

Store-bought soups (low-sodium varieties are still high when you look at the numbers on the label) and soups in restaurants or at salad bars

Frozen dinners

Most, but not *all,* restaurant food (Chefs *love* to pour on salt to increase flavor. I know this firsthand, as about a decade ago I owned a firm called At Home Chef and watched the chefs work their magic with a heavy dose of salt.)

Canned products (I eat white albacore tuna but always rinse it in a strainer before eating.)

Salty snacks, such as chips (Why do you think their name starts with the word "salt"?)

Vegetable juice and Bloody Mary mix (a killer when it comes to sodium content; check out the label if you don't believe me)

Soy and teriyaki sauces

2. **Exercise.** The more you exercise and the more intensely you exercise (you will soon learn that intensity is your BFF when it comes to optimizing metabolism) will cause you to lose more water through both perspiration and breathing. A study conducted by trainer Amanda Carlson found that 98 percent of football players preparing for a major scouting event were dehydrated in the morning when they began their first evaluation. She goes on to state that "just losing 2 percent of your body weight in fluid can decrease performance by up to 25 percent."[6] It should also be noted that dehydration slows the recovery process postexercise. We actually want to speed up this process, so always maintaining an acceptable water balance is clearly a *REVVED* behavior.

3. **Climate.** When I am in the desert in the likes of Palm Springs or Las Vegas, I notice I immediately need to drink more water because of the dry air. Ditto in the cold winters in Chicago when the dry heat is blazing. I am a humidifier junkie and have them everywhere—my home, office, you name it—as I notice that dry air dehydrates me quickly.

4. **Medication.** Certain medication, such as diuretics or "water pills," which are sometimes prescribed for high blood pressure, kidney and liver problems, and heart failure, to name a few, work by flushing unneeded water and salt out through your urine. These may require more or even less water. When I take my son, Evan, to an amusement park and he implores me to go on rides that I have *no* business going on (because they both petrify me and make me sick), I take antinausea medication. I'm terribly dehydrated as a result and find myself having to drink a ton of extra water.

Eat Water-Rich Foods

It's true, you can both drink *and* eat water. Not only are foods high in water content hydrating but they also fill you up and cause you to eat less higher-calorie food throughout the day. Why? Because these hydrating foods are vegetables and fruit, and I've already preached the enormous benefits of these *REVVED* foods when it comes to their high fiber content, their beneficial effect on blood sugar, and so on.

Here is a list of some of the best water-rich foods, which you will be frequently eating during your 28-day *REVVED* Eating Plan, and I hope forevermore:

Vegetables that are 90 percent or more water include

Bell pepper	Eggplant
Broccoli	Spinach
Celery	Tomato
Cucumber	Zucchini

Fruits that are 85 percent or more water include

Blueberries	Pineapple
Cantaloupe	Strawberries
Grapefruit	Watermelon[7]
Oranges	

Tea

Tea is a powerful part of the *REVVED* plan. Let's start with what many researchers consider the "gold standard" when it comes to tea. That designation goes to green tea.

Green Tea

Green tea is believed to be more powerful than some of its "sister" teas, because it does not go through the fermentation process that, say, black tea does. By not going through fermentation, green tea retains the highest concentration of powerful antioxidants called polyphenols.

Green tea has many benefits. Among them are that it:

1. **Helps you lose weight.** Green tea contains a bounty of powerful antioxidants, one of which is called EGCG, or epigallocatechin gallate. EGCG, coupled with the caffeine that is found in green tea, speeds up weight loss by stimulating your metabolism. Caffeine alone can accomplish this metabolic boost, but coupling it with EGCG makes it much more powerful. Most research studies estimate the number of additional calories burned by drinking green tea to be 70 to 100 a day.

2. **Burns fat.** The combination of EGCG and caffeine also stimulates the release of fat into the bloodstream so that, instead of being stored, the fat gets used for fuel. The combination of EGCG and caffeine can actually help to dissolve fat in the bloodstream. Triglycerides are what sugar and fat are synthesized into. Triglycerides get a bad rap but shouldn't, as they are an important substance that supplies energy to numerous functions in the body. They should get a bad rap only when there are too many circulating, making you run the risk of their being stored in your cells as body fat. Green tea's large number of polyphenols are also good for weight loss, as they activate an enzyme that literally dissolves the triglycerides that aren't going to be used. In essence, drinking green tea gobbles them up, like that little Pac-Man I talked about earlier. Gobbling up excess fat is very good for a *REVVED* body.

3. **Enhances energy.** Let's face it, you need a little more energy. You can get that from green tea, and that extra energy will be perfect for those days you perform your interval-based strength training.

4. **Repairs muscle.** By now you know you will be creating microscopic tears in your muscle through strength training. If you can repair those muscles faster, you can lift heavier and enhance metabolism that much more. I just mentioned that staying properly hydrated helps repair muscle, but my personal experience with drinking more green tea agrees with the research that drinking it enhances accelerated repair even more.[8]

In addition to these clear benefits, green tea has been shown to:

Reduce the rise of heart disease and stroke

Lower LDL, the bad cholesterol, and raise HDL, the good cholesterol

Lower the risk of numerous cancers

Enable blood sugar to remain at more appropriate levels (a fasting, first-think-in-the-morning blood-sugar level is optimally 70 to 100 milligrams per deciliter), which benefits both type 1 and type 2 diabetics

Stave off liver disease

Reduce inflammation (*Note:* Inflammation, or an excess amount of inflammation, dramatically accelerates the aging process. Inflammation crushes a *REVVED* opportunity. We don't want it, and I will teach you how to avoid it.)

Other Teas

Here is a list of lesser-known teas and some of their beneficial properties:

1. **Pu-erh tea.** Pu-erh tea is actually made from the same leaves and stems as those used for green, oolong, and black teas, from the *Camellia sinensis* plant. As I mentioned, green tea is not fermented. Pu-erh tea is fermented, but then it is aged under high humidity to make it taste better. The specific benefits of pu-erh include the following:

    It lowers LDL, the bad cholesterol, and raises HDL, the good.

    It may gobble up triglycerides, and therefore shrink fat cells.

    Dr. Oz strongly believes in pu-erh and recommends that you consume 2 cups each morning with your breakfast.

2. **White tea.** White tea possesses properties very similar to those of green tea. White tea leaves are not fermented, but they are picked earlier, which leads some researchers to believe that, of all the teas, white tea may actually be the most potent. The issue is that, in the past, white tea was not as available as green or black tea was, but that appears to be changing, as food companies are jumping on the white-tea bandwagon, and the proliferation of boutique tea stores has made white tea more accessible.

    One study on white tea caught my eye. According to researcher Milton Schiffenbauer, a microbiologist and professor at Pace University, "Past studies have shown that green tea stimulates the immune system to fight disease. Our research shows white tea extract can actually destroy in vitro the organisms that cause disease."[9] The ability to destroy organisms is pretty powerful. I'll stay tuned for more press on white tea, but in the meantime I've added it to my tea rotation.

3. **Black tea.** When you drink traditional iced tea, which I pound all the time, you are consuming black tea. Although it is fermented, and therefore contains fewer antioxidants than white or green tea, it is

still an excellent choice, as it remains very high on the antioxidant scoreboard. As well as adding lemon to water, I add lemon to every single glass of tea I drink. I frequently ask for more lemon and squeeze away. I also find that adding lemon to my black tea does not necessitate adding any artificial sweetener, sugar, or honey.

For that matter, all of the teas I am recommending are in their pure form. I do not add milk or any type of sweetener. If you are used to drinking tea with some type of sweetener, then I urge you to wean yourself off of it. If you use one packet, start using a half packet. Just sprinkle a little in and remember, the lemon will also add a lot of flavor.

Sports Drinks, Soda, and Juice

Let me be very clear: No, no, and no! Let's take these disasters one at a time.

Sports Drinks

Sports drinks, at 8 calories an ounce, are a complete and utter marketing sham. The only time you need a sports drink is when you are in the twenty-first mile of a marathon, which you will learn in chapter 7 should never be done, as people die during marathons, or if you are in the final set at Wimbledon. Don't believe the line that you need to "replace electrolytes" or any other part of the marketing propaganda put out by sports-drink companies. If you are engaging in a long-duration sport, have the correct snack on hand and skip the useless, expensive sports drinks. Moms and dads, this is especially important for kids. Just say NO to sports drinks in the house—or anywhere, for that matter.

Soda

Soda is another disaster at 12 calories an ounce. Take a look at this data: "A Yale University Rudd Center for Food Policy and Obesity study found that a majority of Americans understand that soda is bad for them. But despite this, a Gallup poll reveals that 48 percent of surveyed Americans—nearly half!—drink soda on a daily basis. What's more, among those who drank soda, the average daily intake was 2.6 glasses per day."[10]

That intake of 2.6 glasses is probably 26 ounces, as you have to assume 10-ounce and not 8-ounce glasses, since the size of most glasses has increased substantially. Therefore, that 26 ounces times 12 calories per ounce equals 312 soda calories a day.

According to Dr. Mark Hyman, high-fructose corn syrup, the sweetener found in most sodas, "is absorbed more rapidly than regular sugar, and it doesn't stimulate insulin or leptin production. This prevents you from triggering the body's signals for being full and may lead to overconsumption of total calories."[11]

When you first read about soda, you probably assumed it was mostly kids and teens who were drinking it. But I'm shocked—no, appalled—when I sit next to affluent, well-dressed individuals on the plane who, at 8:00 P.M. flying home out of LaGuardia, order a soda. Frequently they drink more than one. What's that about? Don't they know they are drinking liquid poison, often with caffeine? They will be so surprised when they are still wide awake at 1:30 A.M. They disrupted not only their sleep but also their hormones and their ability to optimally produce human growth hormone. It's a disastrous choice.

This same type of person will sit next to me at a dinner party and proclaim, "I just don't know why I can't lose weight and why I feel exhausted all the time." It's because they *told* their body to feel that way.

Juice

I kept juice for last on purpose, as it is the absolute worst possible form of liquid calories that can ever pass your lips. It's evil. It's 15 calories an ounce, so it packs a greater caloric punch than the first two. The reason I get so amped up about juice (and not in a positive way) is that we are barraged with advertisements that proclaim all the antioxidant benefits of juice, with its nutrients and vitamins such as C. It's all such a sham.

Juice is pasteurized. That means that, for a short period of time, it is heated to a high temperature. Pasteurization is beneficial, because it destroys molds, bacteria, and other unwanted microorganisms that might be in the juice. Juice manufacturers aren't sure those things truly are in there. They are just doing it to be safe. Pasteurization also prolongs shelf life, which is a primary goal of many food and juice manufacturers.

But heating the juice to a high temperature, even for a short period of time, also does one more thing: It eradicates, or more specifically incinerates, the vitamins, minerals, and enzymes and leaves only sugar water. Not good.

So all the hype about the benefits of juice is just that—hype. Here's another one of my favorites. A deep red juice recently became very popular. On the bottom of the label on the bottle it says that this berry "contains more antioxidants than any other fruit." Oops, did I read "fruit"? I thought this was juice. It's interesting that the manufacturer used the research on the *fruit*, not the *juice*, in its claim on the label.

Let's make a pact: No juice, not ever, not even if you juice it at home.

"Wait," you must be thinking. "Why can't I make my own juice at home? I won't pasteurize it. I will just make it and drink it."

The problem with that goes back to a word I introduced you to very early on: "satiety." Here's the research:

Dr. Richard Mattes, of Purdue University, conducted an experiment in which he compared the difference in calorie consumption between one group who ate a lunch of solid foods and a second group who ate the exact same lunch (with the same calories, protein, carbohydrates, fat, and fiber) in liquid form. They were all then allowed to eat whatever they wanted for the rest of the day. The researchers found that the liquid-lunch drinkers ate 12 to 19 percent more food during the rest of the day than the solid-food eaters.[12]

Mattes and his team conducted a second study, this time analyzing the response of the participants to three forms of the same food. Group 1 got a whole apple, group 2 got applesauce, and group 3 got apple juice (calorie counts were the same). Group 3, the apple-juice drinkers, had the greatest hunger afterward. Group 1, the whole-apple eaters, had the least amount of hunger, and group 2, the applesauce eaters, fell somewhere in between.[13]

In the jelly bean study, which is one of my favorites, group 1 ate 450 calories of jelly beans and group 2 drank 450 calories of soda each day for a month. The jelly bean eaters reduced their daily caloric intake by about 450 calories, because their body said to them "I'm full," whereas the soda drinkers did not because their bodies paid no attention to the 450 liquid calories consumed.[14]

Wait, I have one more study to share. The Harvard Nurses' Health study of fifty thousand women conducted over eight years found that switching from one sugary drink a *week* to one or more a *day* resulted in 358 more calories consumed per day, and a lot of weight gain.[15]

All of these studies point the same conclusion: Liquid calories don't trigger satiety mechanisms. If you look at all the conclusions, each study found that all or some of the following occurs when people consume calories in liquid form:

> They miss out on the benefits of chewing, which appears to help trigger satiety mechanisms.

> Liquid travels faster through the stomach and intestine than solids.

Ghrelin, the hunger hormone, is generally turned off when the stomach stretches with solid food. Since liquids do not expand the stomach, ghrelin does not turn off and, instead, keeps pumping out and asking, "Where's the food?"

In addition to ghrelin, other hormones that trigger satiety in the stomach are not turned on when calories are consumed in liquid form.

It's also theorized that liquid, which is so fast and easy to drink, doesn't give people the psychological feeling that they are taking in calories. It's as if the liquid calories "don't get any respect," so the mind ignores them and keeps searching for more calories.

Richard Mattes, a researcher involved in two of the studies above, sums it up beautifully when he says, "Fluid calories do not hold strong satiety properties, don't suppress hunger, and don't elicit compensatory dietary responses. In fact, when drinking fluid calories, people often end up eating more calories overall."[16]

Therefore, let's be clear. You are not going to consume liquid calories of any kind. The only exception will be your whey-protein breakfast shake and your *REVVED* soup. Thicker shakes, which contain protein and fruit, require more time to drink, fill up the stomach, efficiently turn on and off your hormones to trigger satiety, and take far longer (because of the fiber content in fruit) to pass through the stomach and intestines. Therefore, they are an exception—of course you have to be drinking the right type of shake (more on that later).

Coffee

I have also eliminated from the *REVVED* Eating Plan all liquid calories masquerading as coffee. I'm sorry, but a 500-calorie coffee drink, and we all know what I'm talking about, is a disaster to your *REVVED* aspirations. It's pure sugar and nutritionally devoid of any nutrients and vitamins. Okay, the small amount of low-fat milk is fine, but the rest is chocolate shavings, butterscotch topping, and whipped cream. *Really*, is that any way to start your day or give yourself an afternoon pick-me-up? Those drinks shut you down, because they put you on both the sugar and the caffeine highways. By that, I mean we know the quick, empty sugar will result in a sugar party that gets shut down by insulin. Translation? You crash.

Ditto with too much caffeine. Most of those drinks are made with triple-power espresso beans, so you get a crazed caffeine rush. What does your smart body think about that? "No, thank you," it says and sends hormones to calm you down. You just lost the extra pep that intelligent caffeine, such as that in the teas I have recommended, gives you. Regular coffee in the proper portion size is fine. But keep it to 1 to 2 cups a day.

Alcohol

Okay, let's cover the final liquid calorie, alcohol. A truth: I love wine. Another truth: I also love the occasional martini, either gin or vodka. And most of my clients love some form of alcohol and embrace the social aspects of this favorite liquid calorie. So what's our strategy with alcohol?

First, let's talk calories. Generally, wine is 20 to 25 calories an ounce, so that a 5-ounce glass of white wine with dinner is 100 calories. If the wine is red (which is generally higher in proof), it will be about 125 calories.

Hard liquor calories go up with proof. The higher the proof, the higher the calorie count per ounce:

70 proof vodka, which is 35 percent alcohol, contains 55 calories.

80 proof vodka, which is 40 percent alcohol, contains 65 calories.

90 proof vodka, which is 45 percent alcohol, contains 75 calories.

In this 28-day *REVVED* plan, I have eliminated alcohol. There—I said it. Allow that to sink in. I'm bringing your calories down to facilitate quick weight and fat loss, and I simply do not feel there is room for alcohol. I also want you to optimize how great you are going to feel on this plan and not disrupt your sleep cycle, as alcohol has been shown to do, depending on the amount you drink and the time you consume it. So let's just agree to take a 28-day break from alcohol.

But if, when those 28 days are over, you decide there is some room to include alcohol in your ongoing *REVVED* plan, then please heed this advice: *Always be a two-fisted drinker.* By that I mean consume 2 ounces of water for every ounce of alcohol. This will help you in three ways:

1. **You will probably drink less, because you are filling up on water.** In chapter 5, you learned that drinking 2 glasses of water before breakfast helped people reach satiety, so they ate less. The same will hold true with drinking water with your alcohol, as you will drink less.

2. **You will feel *so much better* in the morning.** Alcohol robs the body of water, because it breaks down while you are sleeping. If you start ahead of the game and drink lots of water the night before, your body has more residual water to use, and you will therefore wake up less dehydrated than if you only drank alcoholic drinks.

3. **You will look *so much better* in the morning.** Again, that smart body of yours feels your water levels are getting low and wonders, "Are we stuck somewhere without a proper supply of water? I'm worried and am therefore going to hold on to all my reserves." By drinking lots of water both at night and then in the morning, you send the opposite signal, "Release the reserves," and you will lose the water bloat. You will like the way you look and feel when that happens.

A note to frequent fliers: You lose a tremendous amount of water on the plane as a result of dry cabin air. Most of the time, we exist in air that is 40 to 70 percent humidity, but the air inside a plane, on account of cabin pressure, falls to 20 percent humidity, so please make it a point to drink water before, during, and after a flight. Who wants to start an exciting or demanding business trip with a pounding headache from dehydration?

The Diet Drink Dilemma

I have to be honest; I used to be a diet drink–aholic. I drank 100 to 150 ounces daily. I pounded it from morning until night. Then, around seven years ago, I woke up and said, "That's it. I'm done," and have never had a sip since.

There is some compelling research against diet beverages in general. Lyn M. Steffen, associate professor of epidemiology at the University of Minnesota, found that the risk of metabolic syndrome, defined as the "triple threat" of high blood pressure, high cholesterol, and high blood sugar, increased a full 34 percent in those who consumed just one, and only one, diet soda a day.[17] Sharon P. Fowler and colleagues at the University of Texas Health Science Center studied fifteen hundred people between the ages of twenty-five and fifty-four and found that for each can of diet soda they consumed, their risk of obesity shot up by 41 percent.[18]

What's this all about? It's about diet soda. There are a few theories as to why it has such an effect on the body.

One is that artificial sweeteners light up the brain in such a way that those consuming these artificial sweeteners then want more of the real thing and might reach for that cookie, piece of cake, or handful of candy. Researchers at Purdue witnessed that rats fed artificial sweeteners consistently ate more sweets.[19]

Another theory, similar to one I will introduce to you with regard to excessive cardiovascular exercise, is that once individuals consume an artificially sweetened drink, they think, "You know, I was so good—I had the diet rather than sugared soda. I should treat myself."

My advice? Keep diet drinks to the bare minimum, cut their consumption in half, and, over time, try to cut them out completely. I told you to do that when I was discussing iced tea. You have simply gotten used to the taste. Or do what I did. Just go cold turkey. It's up to you, but there has to be something behind that compelling research about the dangers of metabolic syndrome and an increase in obesity in people who drink as little as one diet soda per day. Let's listen to the research, and let's be smart. Better yet, let's *REV*erse that old belief system that artificial sweeteners are fine and back that up with a new behavior: avoiding them!

The REVVED Eating Plan

The *REVVED* Eating Plan will leave you feeling energized and satisfied. Absolutely no starving—ever! Before diving in, please read through the "Getting Started" guide and the grocery lists. Make notes and substitutions as necessary. There are both vegetarian and gluten-free options listed with each recipe, so make sure to update the grocery lists as needed. Please note that some recipes require more prep than others. However, I've also included quick 5- to 10-minute meals to accommodate those with the busiest of schedules. They are tagged "quick meal."

To craft this 28-day eating plan, I enlisted the help of registered dietitian and nutritionist, Juliette Britton, a self-proclaimed foodie and home chef. When she's not seeing clients or giving nutrition workshops, you can find her in the kitchen transforming favorite recipes to healthier (but still delicious) versions . . . all while caring for two young children. Instead of the usual, often boring "grilled chicken and vegetables," I asked Juliette to create tasty, easy-to-prepare, nutritionally dense meals according to the specifications I outlined in chapter 4.

The meal plan starts on Sunday, as it is the primary prep day, but feel free to start on whatever day makes the most sense to you. Just remember that this is a 28-day plan, so pick accordingly.

With any meal plan, please remember the following:

- Cook all meats, eggs, and poultry thoroughly to avoid food-borne illness.

- Store leftovers in airtight containers (preferably glass) and place them in your refrigerator as soon as possible.

- Keep raw meats, poultry, and fish separate from cooked and uncooked foods to avoid cross-contamination.

- Always wash produce thoroughly before consuming, and that includes any organic produce you choose to purchase. Don't think that just because it's organic, it doesn't require a thorough cleaning.

- Enjoy your food! Chew slowly, be mindful of the food you are eating, sit down at your kitchen or dining-room table (please don't eat standing up), and listen to calm, *relaxing* music.

Getting Started

Please check your pantry for the following items. They are common ingredients in a well-stocked kitchen, but add them to your grocery list if needed.

Dry Spices

Basil	Garlic powder
Chili powder	Onion powder
Cinnamon (ground)	Oregano
Crushed red pepper	Paprika
Cumin (ground)	Parsley
Dill	Pumpkin pie spice
Fennel seed (whole)	Rosemary (whole)

Condiments, Seasonings, and Oils

Almond butter

Apple cider vinegar

Balsamic vinegar

Butter (unsalted, from grass-fed cows)

Cocoa powder (unsweetened)

Coconut oil

Cooking spray (olive oil)

Dijon mustard

Honey

Maple syrup (100 percent grade B)

100 percent extra-virgin olive oil

Salt

Soy sauce (reduced sodium)

Grocery Guide: Rather than buying an entire set of dried herbs and spices, check out the bulk section of your grocery store. You can get small amounts of herbs without investing in a full jar. Furthermore, it prevents an over-abundance of rarely used spice jars in the kitchen cupboards!

Kitchen Gadgets

Aside from the typical kitchen equipment, these gadgets will make your life much easier over these 28 days!

1. **Microplane grater:** This nifty tool helps grate ginger and citrus fruits in a snap.

2. **Slow cooker:** No need to get fancy; an inexpensive slow cooker does the trick. This appliance is perfect for preparing *REVVED* Chicken Bone Broth.

3. **Parchment paper:** Who likes to do dishes? Instead, line baking sheets with parchment paper for an easy and quick cleanup. Just make sure not to use it in an oven above 425°F.

4. **Kitchen scale:** In the beginning, it is helpful to weigh your food, so you can get a sense of appropriate portion sizes. It also minimizes the need for measuring cups and spoons . . . which means fewer dishes!

5. **Glass storageware with secure lids:** Get an inexpensive but well-made set of glass containers, preferably one with tight-fitting lids and bottoms and lids that stack, so they take up little room. They will keep food fresher longer and prevent spoilage, so in the long run you end up saving food *and* money.

MENU: Weeks 1 and 3

SUNDAY

Breakfast: Protein-Packed Yogurt Parfait with Almonds and Berries
Lunch: Tuna Salad with Pita "Chips" and Carrot Sticks
Dinner: Roasted Chicken with Broccoli, Tomato, and Rice Medley
Snack: Banana with Almond Butter

MONDAY

Breakfast: Nutty Apple Oatmeal and Breakfast Sausage
Lunch: Tarragon Chicken Salad Boats
Dinner: Thai Turkey Lettuce Wraps
Snack: Veggies with Hummus and Fruit

TUESDAY

Breakfast: The *Classic* Breakfast
Lunch: Shrimp with Jicama and Mango Salad
Dinner: Sundried Tomato, Feta, and Spinach Chicken Salad
Snack: Dill Dip with Pita "Chips" and Veggies

WEDNESDAY

Breakfast: Smoked Salmon Flatbread
Lunch: Grab-and-Go Lunch
Dinner: *REVVED*-Up Soup
Snack: Jicama and Mango Salad

THURSDAY

Breakfast: Mediterranean Breakfast Sandwich and Fruit
Lunch: *REVVED*-Up Soup
Dinner: Parmesan Tilapia with Sundried Tomatoes and Green Beans Almondine
Snack: Spiced Garbanzo Bites

FRIDAY

Breakfast: Chorizo Breakfast Burrito and Melon
Lunch: Honey-Mustard Turkey Pita Pocket
Dinner: Savory Maple-Glazed Salmon with Roasted Rosemary Butternut Squash and Steamed Broccoli
Snack: Spiced Garbanzo Bites

SATURDAY

Breakfast: Chocolate-Banana Protein Shake
Lunch: Mediterranean Salad
Dinner: Cumin-Spiced Flank Steak with Roasted Sweet Potato and Sautéed Veggies
Snack: Cantaloupe and Greek Yogurt

MENU: Weeks 2 and 4

SUNDAY

Breakfast: Turkey and Sweet Potato Hash
Lunch: Flank Steak Salad
Dinner: Spicy Southwest Chicken Sandwich with Veggies
Snack: Guacamole and Veggies

MONDAY

Breakfast: Triple-B Protein Shake
Lunch: The *REVVED* Chicken Spinach Salad
Dinner: Maple-Mustard Pork Loin with Roasted Butternut Squash Puree
Snack: Spicy Dipping Sauce and Veggies

TUESDAY

Breakfast: The *REVVED* Omelet
Lunch: Turkey Roll-Up
Dinner: *REVVED* Creamy Chicken Tortilla Soup
Snack: Cheesy Garlic Kale Chips

WEDNESDAY

Breakfast: Oatmeal Ambrosia
Lunch: *REVVED* Creamy Chicken Tortilla Soup
Dinner: Turkey Eggplant Parmesan
Snack: Tomato and Cucumber Crackers

THURSDAY

Breakfast: Grain-Free Banana-Blueberry Pancakes
Lunch: Egg Salad
Dinner: Shrimp Tacos with Pineapple Salsa
Snack: Turkey, Apple, and Cheese "Sandwich"

FRIDAY

Breakfast: Whipped Cottage Cheese with Fruit and Nuts
Lunch: *REVVED* Hawaiian Pizza
Dinner: Seared Sea Scallops with Roasted Garlic Potatoes and Green Beans
Snack: Black Bean and Pineapple Salad

SATURDAY

Breakfast: On-the-Go Breakfast
Lunch: Portobello Mushroom and Spinach Dip with Pita "Chips"
Dinner: *REVVVED* Turkey Casserole
Snack: Whipped Cottage Cheese with Fruit and Nuts

GROCERY LIST: 1,200-Calorie Meal Plan, Week 1

Denotes items you can freeze to last you the entire meal plan.

PRODUCE

3 lemons
3 limes
1 apple
1½ cups seedless grapes
½ cantaloupe or
    1½ cups cubed
1 banana
1 half pint blueberries
1 pint strawberries
1 mango
1 half pint cherry
    tomatoes
3 tomatoes
1 yellow bell pepper
4 red bell peppers
1 jalapeño (optional)
4 carrots
1 10-ounce bag shredded
    carrots
1 cucumber
1 head celery
1 head romaine lettuce
10 ounces baby spinach
1 medium jicama
1 large sweet potato
1 yellow onion
2 red onions
1 head garlic
1 small knob gingerroot
1 bunch fresh parsley
1 bunch fresh cilantro
Fresh dill
Fresh basil
Fresh tarragon

OILS, NUTS, AND SEEDS

1 cup slivered almonds*

FROZEN FOODS

30 ounces broccoli
20 ounces butternut
    squash
20 ounces green beans

MEAT, POULTRY, AND FISH

1 rotisserie chicken
1 (6-count) package
    chicken breakfast
    sausage* (100 calories
    each)
3 ounces wild smoked
    salmon
4 ounces wild salmon
7 ounces sliced turkey
    luncheon meat
3½ ounces shrimp
12 ounces 93 percent lean
    ground turkey
2½ ounces chorizo (about
    1 sausage link)
6 ounces tilapia or cod
9 ounces flank steak
1 3-ounce can light tuna
    packed in water

DAIRY/REFRIGERATOR

1 small container hummus
2 cups 2 percent milk
30 ounces 2 percent plain
    Greek yogurt
1 small container whipped
    cream cheese
2½ ounces feta cheese
6 large eggs
⅓ cup shredded Parmesan
    cheese

GROCERY

1 cup brown rice
5 ounces old-fashioned
    oats
1 small jar sundried
    tomatoes packed in
    olive oil
1 14½-ounce can fire-
    roasted tomatoes
1 14½-ounce can white
    beans
1 14½-ounce can
    garbanzo beans
1 small jar pitted olives
1 tub whey protein
    powder
1 (6-count) package
    sprouted whole-grain
    tortillas*
1 (6-count) package
    sprouted whole-grain
    English muffins*
1 (6-count) package
    sprouted whole-grain
    pitas (100 calories/
    each)*

GROCERY LIST: 1,200-Calorie Meal Plan, Week 2

*Denotes items you can freeze to last you the entire meal plan.

PRODUCE

3 apples
2 bananas
1 pear
1 nectarine, peach, or plum
1 pint strawberries
1 lemon
3 limes
1 clementine
1¼ cups cubed pineapple
1 pint cherry tomatoes
3 tomatoes
1 yellow bell pepper
2 red bell peppers
4 carrots
1 large cucumber
1 eggplant
1 large zucchini
1 head romaine lettuce
10 ounces baby spinach
8 to 10 ounces kale
2 sweet potatoes
1 small potato
1 portobello mushroom
1 yellow onion
1 red onion
1 bunch fresh cilantro
Fresh basil
4 2-ounce guacamole* minis (100-calorie portions)

OILS, NUTS, AND SEEDS

½ cup raw whole almonds*
⅓ cup raw pecan pieces*
1 tablespoon pine nuts*
⅓ cup raw walnut pieces*

FROZEN FOODS

2 cups blueberries*

MEAT, POULTRY, AND FISH

1 rotisserie chicken
5 ounces sliced turkey luncheon meat
6 ounces shrimp
8 ounces sea scallops
9 ounces 93 percent lean ground turkey
4 ounces boneless pork loin

DAIRY/REFRIGERATOR

2 cups 2 percent milk
30 ounces 2 percent plain Greek yogurt
2 cups 2 percent cottage cheese
2 ounces goat cheese
1 dozen large eggs
¾ cup shredded Parmesan cheese

GROCERY

1 7-ounce can chipotle peppers in adobo sauce*
1 10-ounce can diced tomatoes with green chilis
1 14-ounce can tomato sauce
1 14½-ounce can black beans
1 small package woven wheat crackers (such as Triscuits)
1 small container nutritional yeast
¾ cup raisins
1 (6-count) package 6-inch corn tortillas*

GROCERY LIST: 1,200-Calorie Meal Plan, Week 3

*Denotes items you can freeze to last you the entire meal plan.

PRODUCE

3 lemons
3 limes
1 apple
1½ cups seedless grapes
½ cantaloupe or 1½ cups cubed
1 banana
1 half pint blueberries
1 pint strawberries
1 mango
1 half pint cherry tomatoes
3 tomatoes
1 yellow bell pepper
4 red bell peppers
1 jalapeño (optional)
4 carrots
1 10-ounce bag shredded carrots
1 cucumber
1 head celery
1 head romaine lettuce
10 ounces baby spinach
1 medium jicama
1 large sweet potato
1 yellow onion
2 red onions
1 head garlic
1 small knob gingerroot
1 bunch fresh parsley
1 bunch fresh cilantro
Fresh dill
Fresh basil
Fresh tarragon

FROZEN FOODS

30 ounces broccoli
20 ounces butternut squash
20 ounces green beans

MEAT, POULTRY, AND FISH

1 rotisserie chicken
3 ounces wild smoked salmon
4 ounces wild salmon
7 ounces sliced turkey luncheon meat
3½ ounces shrimp
12 ounces 93 percent lean ground turkey
2½ ounces chorizo (only if not using frozen burrito from Week 1)
6 ounces tilapia or cod
1 9-ounce flank steak
1 3-ounce can light tuna packed in water

DAIRY/REFRIGERATOR

1 small container hummus
2 cups 2 percent milk
30 ounces 2 percent plain Greek yogurt
1 small container whipped cream cheese
2½ ounces feta cheese
6 large eggs
⅓ cup shredded Parmesan cheese

GROCERY

1 14½-ounce can fire-roasted tomatoes
1 14½-ounce can white beans
1 14½-ounce can garbanzo beans
1 (6-count) package sprouted whole-grain pitas (100 calories/each)
1 (6-count) package sprouted whole-grain tortillas

Denotes items you can freeze to last you the entire meal plan.

PRODUCE

3 apples
2 bananas
1 pear
1 nectarine, peach, or plum
1 pint strawberries
1 lemon
3 limes
1 clementine
1¼ cups pineapple, cubed
1 pint cherry tomatoes
3 tomatoes
1 yellow bell pepper
2 red bell peppers
4 carrots
1 large cucumber
1 large zucchini
1 eggplant
1 head romaine lettuce
10 ounces baby spinach
8 to 10 ounces kale
2 sweet potatoes
1 small potato
1 portobello mushroom
1 yellow onion
1 red onion
1 bunch fresh cilantro
Fresh basil

MEAT, POULTRY, AND FISH

1 rotisserie chicken
5 ounces sliced turkey luncheon meat
6 ounces shrimp
8 ounces sea scallops
9 ounces 93 percent lean ground turkey
4 ounces boneless pork loin

DAIRY/REFRIGERATOR

2 cups 2 percent milk
30 ounces 2 percent plain Greek yogurt*
2 cups 2 percent cottage cheese*
2 ounces goat cheese
1 dozen large eggs
¾ cup shredded Parmesan cheese

GROCERY

1 10-ounce can diced tomatoes with green chilis
1 14½-ounce can tomato sauce
1 14½-ounce can black beans

GROCERY LIST: 1,600-Calorie Meal Plan, Week 1

Denotes items you can freeze to last you the entire meal plan.

PRODUCE

4 lemons
5 limes
1 orange
2 apples
1 cup seedless grapes
½ cantaloupe or 2 cups cubed
1 banana
1 pint blueberries
1 pint strawberries
2 mangos
1 pint cherry tomatoes
3 tomatoes
1 yellow bell pepper
5 red bell peppers
1 jalapeño (optional)
5 carrots
1 10-ounce bag shredded carrots
1 cucumber
1 head celery
1 head romaine lettuce
10 ounces baby spinach
1 large jicama
1 large sweet potato
1 yellow onion
2 red onions
1 head garlic
1 small knob gingerroot
1 bunch fresh parsley
1 bunch fresh cilantro
Fresh dill
Fresh basil
Fresh tarragon

OILS, NUTS, AND SEEDS

1 cup slivered almonds*

FROZEN FOODS

35 ounces broccoli
30 ounces butternut squash
25 ounces green beans

MEAT, POULTRY, AND FISH

1 rotisserie chicken
1 (6-count) package chicken breakfast sausage (100 calories each)*
4 ounces wild smoked salmon
5½ ounces wild salmon
11 ounces sliced turkey luncheon meat
5 ounces shrimp
13½ ounces 93 percent lean ground turkey
3 ounces chorizo (about 1 sausage link)
8 ounces tilapia or cod
1 11-ounce flank steak
1 5-ounce can light tuna packed in water

DAIRY/REFRIGERATOR

1 small container hummus
2 cups 2 percent milk
30 ounces 2 percent Greek yogurt
1 small container whipped cream cheese
3½ ounces feta cheese
1 dozen large eggs
⅓ cup shredded Parmesan cheese

GROCERY

1 cup brown rice
5 ounces old-fashioned oats
1 small jar sundried tomatoes packed in olive oil
1 14½-ounce can fire-roasted tomatoes
1 14½-ounce can white beans
2 14½-ounce cans garbanzo beans
1 small jar pitted olives
1 tub whey protein powder
1 (6-count) package sprouted whole-grain tortillas*
1 (6-count) package sprouted whole-grain English muffins*
2 (6-count) packages sprouted whole-grain pitas (100 calories each)*
1 loaf sprouted whole-grain bread

GROCERY LIST: 1,600-Calorie Meal Plan, Week 2

*Denotes items you can freeze to last you the entire meal plan.

PRODUCE

3 apples
2 bananas
1 pear
1 nectarine, peach, or plum
1 pint strawberries
1 lemon
3 limes
1 orange
1 clementine
1¼ cups cubed pineapple
1½ pints cherry tomatoes
2 tomatoes
2 yellow bell peppers
2 red bell peppers
4 carrots
1 10-ounce bag shredded carrots
1 large cucumber
1 large zucchini
1 eggplant
1 head romaine lettuce
10 ounces baby spinach
8 to 10 ounces kale
2 sweet potatoes
1 small potato
1 portobello mushroom
1 yellow onion
1 red onion
1 bunch fresh cilantro
Fresh basil
4 2-ounce guacamole minis (100-calorie portions)*

OILS, NUTS, AND SEEDS

½ cup raw whole almonds*
⅓ cup raw pecan pieces*
1 tablespoon raw pine nuts*
⅓ cup raw walnut pieces*

FROZEN FOODS

10 to 12 ounces blueberries*

MEAT, POULTRY, AND FISH

1 rotisserie chicken
8 ounces sliced turkey luncheon meat
7 ounces shrimp
10 ounces sea scallops
12½ ounces 93 percent lean ground turkey
5½ ounces boneless pork loin

DAIRY/REFRIGERATOR

2 cups 2 percent milk
30 ounces 2 percent Greek yogurt
2¾ cups 2 percent cottage cheese
2 ounces goat cheese
1 dozen large eggs
¾ cup shredded Parmesan cheese

GROCERY

1 7-ounce can chipotle peppers in adobo sauce*
1 10-ounce can diced tomatoes with green chilis
1 14½-ounce can tomato sauce
1 14½-ounce can black beans
1 package woven wheat crackers (such as Triscuits)
1 small container nutritional yeast
¾ cup raisins
1 (6-count) package 6-inch corn tortillas*

GROCERY LIST: 1,600-Calorie Meal Plan, Week 3

*Denotes items you can freeze to last you the entire meal plan.

PRODUCE

4 lemons
5 limes
1 orange
2 apples
2 cups seedless grapes
½ cantaloupe or 2 cups cubed
1 banana
1 pint blueberries
1 pint strawberries
2 mangos
1 pint cherry tomatoes
3 tomatoes
1 yellow bell pepper
5 red bell peppers
1 jalapeño (optional)
5 carrots
1 10-ounce bag shredded carrots
1 cucumber
1 head celery
1 head romaine lettuce
10 ounces baby spinach
1 large jicama
1 large sweet potato
1 yellow onion
2 large red onions
1 head garlic
1 small knob gingerroot
1 bunch fresh parsley
1 bunch fresh cilantro
Fresh dill
Fresh basil
Fresh tarragon

FROZEN FOODS

35 ounces broccoli
30 ounces butternut squash
25 ounces green beans

MEAT, POULTRY, AND FISH

1 rotisserie chicken
4 ounces wild smoked salmon
5½ ounces wild salmon
11 ounces sliced turkey luncheon meat
5 ounces shrimp
13 ounces 93 percent lean ground turkey
3 ounces chorizo (only if not using frozen burrito from Week 1)
8 ounces tilapia or cod
1 11-ounce flank steak
1 5-ounce can light tuna packed in water

DAIRY/REFRIGERATOR

1 small container hummus
2 cups 2 percent milk
30 ounces 2 percent Greek yogurt
1 small container whipped cream cheese
3½ ounces feta cheese
1 dozen large eggs
⅓ cup shredded Parmesan cheese

GROCERY

1 14½-ounce can fire-roasted tomatoes
1 14½-ounce can white beans
2 14½-ounce cans garbanzo beans
1 (6-count) package sprouted whole-grain tortillas

Denotes items you can freeze to last you the entire meal plan.

PRODUCE

3 apples
2 bananas
1 pear
1 nectarine, peach, or plum
1 pint strawberries
1 lemon
3 limes
1 orange
1 clementine
1¼ cups cubed pineapple
1½ pints cherry tomatoes
2 tomatoes
2 yellow bell peppers
2 red bell peppers
4 carrots
1 large cucumber
1 large zucchini
1 eggplant
1 head romaine lettuce
10 ounces baby spinach
8 to 10 ounces kale
2 sweet potatoes
1 small potato
1 portobello mushroom
1 yellow onion
1 red onion
1 bunch fresh cilantro
Fresh basil

MEAT, POULTRY, AND FISH

1 rotisserie chicken
8 ounces sliced turkey luncheon meat
7 ounces shrimp
10 ounces sea scallops
12½ ounces 93 percent lean ground turkey
5½ ounces boneless pork loin

DAIRY/REFRIGERATOR

2 cups 2 percent milk
30 ounces 2 percent Greek yogurt
2¾ cups 2 percent cottage cheese
2 ounces goat cheese
1 dozen large eggs
¾ cup shredded Parmesan cheese

GROCERY

1 10-ounce can diced tomatoes with green chilis
1 14½-ounce can tomato sauce
1 14½-ounce can black beans
1 (6-count) package 6-inch corn tortillas
1 (6-count) package sprouted whole-grain pitas (100 calories each)

Substitutions

I want this meal plan to work for you! Here are some substitutions in the event you don't care for a particular ingredient or want to take advantage of seasonal produce. Please note that the substitutions will alter the nutrition profile *slightly*, but it will still be within the *REVVED* nutrition guidelines.

Vegetables

Take your pick of any of the nonstarchy vegetables. Don't like carrots? Swap them out for cauliflower or broccoli. Just make sure to keep portion sizes relatively the same. Here is a short list of nonstarchy veggies to consider: artichoke, asparagus, broccoli, cauliflower, celery, cucumber, eggplant, mushroom, radish, summer squash, tomato, and zucchini.

Fruit

IN PLACE OF . . .	TRY . . .
1 cup grapes	1 plum, peach, or apricot or 2 figs
½ banana	¾ cup chopped watermelon or ½ cup chopped mango
½ cup chopped mango	½ cup chopped papaya or pineapple
1 apple	1 pear, nectarine, or peach
¾ cup sliced strawberries	¾ cup raspberries, blackberries, or blueberries
1 orange	2 clementines or ½ grapefruit

Animal Protein

Please keep portion sizes the same; for example, 4 ounces chicken breast equals 4 ounces pork tenderloin.

IN PLACE OF . . .	TRY . . .
skinless chicken breast	pork tenderloin
salmon	tuna steak
tilapia	cod, barramundi, or halibut
shrimp	scallops or calamari
ground turkey	ground chicken or extra-lean ground beef

Dairy

Nondairy milk alternatives (soy, coconut, almond, etc.) can replace the milk in all of the recipes. However, when compared to 2 percent milk, most of the nondairy alternatives, with the exception of soy, contain 30 to 40 percent fewer calories and 4 to 5 fewer grams of protein per cup. Since the *REVVED* plan has very few recipes with 2 percent milk, there's no need to make meal-plan adjustments. Please be sure to purchase nonsweetened varieties of any nondairy milk alternative.

IN PLACE OF . . .	TRY . . .
Parmesan cheese	mozzarella cheese
feta cheese	goat cheese
whipped cream cheese	goat cheese or Laughing Cow cheese product

Grains

Please keep portion sizes the same.

IN PLACE OF . . .	TRY . . .
brown rice	quinoa, barley, or whole-wheat pasta
English muffin	mini whole-grain bagel or mochi
1 slice bread	5 woven wheat crackers
oatmeal	quinoa, grits, brown rice, or millet

Grocery Guide

Fat-free yogurt? Not so fast. Choose yogurts and other dairy products with moderate amounts of fat to help promote satiety and prevent spikes in blood-glucose levels.

When shopping for canned tuna, opt for the light or skipjack tuna, as they are lower in mercury.

Look for luncheon meat with minimal additives, such as nitrates or nitrites. Trader Joe's, Costco, and major grocery chains offer a variety of *natural* luncheon meats, such as Applegate or Boar's Head.

Butternut squash can be a hassle to cut and prepare. Opt for precut or the frozen variety to cut down on prep time.

When in season, fresh green beans can't be beat. However, frozen green beans may contain more nutrients, as they are picked at optimal times and flash-frozen.

Preshredded carrots are a wonderful and convenient way to add more veggies and texture to your salads, sandwiches, and soups.

Look for 100 percent extra-virgin olive oil in a dark glass bottle. Olive oil is subject to oxidation, so exposure to light and heat can destroy this healthy fat.

Brand Guide

Looking for help choosing specific brands? Here are some of my favorites:

Breakfast sausage: Amylu

Butter: Kerrygold

Canned tuna: Wild Planet

Luncheon meats: Applegate or Boar's Head

Greek yogurt: Fage 2 percent plain

Meat, 100 percent grass-fed and finished: U.S. Wellness Meats, Wallace Farms, Whole Foods

Poultry, 100 percent pasture-raised: U.S. Wellness Meats, Wallace Farms, Whole Foods

Milk: Organic Valley (pastured raised)

Protein powder: MCT Lean

Sprouted breads, pitas, English muffins: Ezekiel

Sprouted wheat tortillas: Maria and Ricardo (gluten-free)

Sprouted corn tortillas: Ezekiel

Sunday BREAKFAST

(quick meal) Protein-Packed Yogurt Parfait with Almonds and Berries

1 cup 2 percent plain Greek yogurt
1 tablespoon almond butter
½ tablespoon honey
½ teaspoon cinnamon or pumpkin pie spice
¾ cup sliced strawberries
2 tablespoons slivered almonds

1. In a medium bowl, mix the yogurt, almond butter, honey, and cinnamon.

2. Top the mixture with the strawberries and slivered almonds.

GLUTEN-FREE SUBSTITUTION: Naturally gluten-free!

NUTRITION TIP: Cinnamon, as little as ½ teaspoon per day, has been shown to help regulate blood-glucose levels and promote insulin sensitivity.[1]

Nutrition information: calories: 410, fat: 21 g., carbs: 34 g., protein: 27 g., fiber: 7 g.

(quick meal) Tuna Salad with Pita "Chips" and Carrot Sticks

1 sprouted whole-grain pita
3 ounces tuna packed in water, drained
2 tablespoons hummus
1 tablespoon lemon juice
1 tablespoon chopped parsley
1 cup carrot sticks

1. Toast the pita; when it is golden brown, slice it into wedges.

2. Drain the tuna well and place it in a small bowl.

3. Add the hummus, lemon juice, and parsley and mix until the salad is incorporated.

4. Serve the tuna salad with pita "chips" and carrot sticks.

GLUTEN-FREE SUBSTITUTION: Serve with gluten-free crackers or a brown-rice tortilla.

VEGETARIAN SUBSTITUTION: Replace the tuna with 2 hard-boiled eggs.

SHORTCUT: Find a flavorful hummus, such as roasted red pepper, and omit the lemon juice and fresh parsley.

NUTRITION TIP: Tuna is an excellent source of DHA and EPA, two omega-3 fatty acids shown to help reduce inflammation and promote heart health and healthy aging.

Nutrition information: calories: 280, fat: 5 g., carbs: 32 g., protein: 29 g., fiber: 6 g.

Sunday DINNER

Roasted Chicken with Broccoli, Tomato, and Rice Medley

1 cup brown rice
1 rotisserie chicken
½ tablespoon lemon juice
2 tablespoons freshly chopped parsley
Salt and pepper to taste
5 cherry tomatoes, halved
1 cup frozen broccoli, steamed
1 tablespoon shredded Parmesan cheese

1. Cook the rice according to its package directions.
2. While the rice cooks, remove the skin from the chicken.
3. Cut the breast meat off both sides and set it aside. (The remainder of the rotisserie chicken will be used later for chicken broth.)
4. When the rice is ready, place ½ cup of the cooked rice in a bowl (store the remainder in the refrigerator for Monday's and Tuesday's dinners).
5. Mix the rice with the lemon juice, parsley, salt, and pepper.
6. Add the tomatoes and steamed broccoli and toss gently.
7. Top with the cheese, and serve with 4 ounces of the chicken breast.

GLUTEN-FREE SUBSTITUTION: Naturally gluten-free!

VEGETARIAN SUBSTITUTION: Replace the chicken with a vegetarian patty, such as a Sunshine Burger.

NUTRITION TIP: Chicken is a lean source of protein filled with good nutrition. If at all possible, choose pastured-raised chickens, which have been shown to have higher amounts of vitamins A and E and up to 25 percent more omega-3s compared to chickens fed an all-grain diet.

STORAGE TIP: Place the remaining chicken breast in an airtight container. Do not cut it into cubes or slices; it will be less likely to dry out when intact. If gelatin forms on the outside of the chicken, simply wipe it off. Make sure to use it within three days from the date of purchase.[2]

Nutrition information: calories: 360, fat: 7 g., carbs: 34 g., protein: 43 g., fiber: 7 g.

REVVED Chicken Bone Broth

This is your own homemade chicken broth! Two cups will be used for the *REVVED*-Up Soup for Wednesday's dinner. Store the remainder in the freezer for future use.

Makes about 3½ cups

> 1 rotisserie chicken (remaining from dinner)
> 5 cups water
> 1 tablespoon apple cider vinegar

1. Remove all the skin from the chicken and discard it.

2. Cut the chicken into pieces.

3. Place all the chicken pieces in a slow cooker.

4. Add the water and vinegar.

5. Cook on low for 7 to 8 hours.

6. Strain the broth and store it in an airtight container in the refrigerator.

NUTRITION TIP: Put down that carton of store-bought broth! Take these simple steps and make your own very healthy and healing bone broth. Bone broth is packed with essential vitamins and minerals, such as calcium, magnesium, and zinc! Next time you're feeling under the weather, make your favorite soup with this simple chicken bone broth recipe.

Sunday SNACK

Banana with Almond Butter

> ½ banana
> 2 teaspoons almond butter

Slice the banana into rounds and top each round with a bit of almond butter.

Nutrition information: calories: 110, fat: 5 g., carbs: 15 g., protein: 3 g., fiber: 3 g.

Nutty Apple Oatmeal and Breakfast Sausage

⅓ cup old-fashioned oats
⅓ cup 2 percent milk
1 tablespoon almond butter
½ small apple, diced
¼ teaspoon cinnamon or pumpkin pie spice (optional)
1 chicken breakfast sausage

1. Cook the oats according to the package directions, using the milk. If you like your oatmeal thinner, add 2 tablespoons of water.

2. When the oatmeal is ready, add the almond butter, diced apple, and cinnamon (save the remaining ½ apple for Wednesday's breakfast).

3. Serve the oatmeal with the chicken sausage.

GLUTEN-FREE SUBSTITUTION: Use gluten-free oats.

VEGETARIAN SUBSTITUTION: Add 2 tablespoons almond butter rather than 1 and omit the chicken sausage.

NUTRITION TIP: Oatmeal is a natural source of plant sterols. Plant sterols have been shown to help reduce cholesterol levels and promote heart health.[3]

STORAGE TIP: Store the remaining ½ apple (unpeeled and unchopped) flesh-side down on a small plate in the fridge, or if you're on the go, place it in an airtight container with a touch of lemon juice to prevent browning.

Nutrition information: calories: 420, fat: 22 g., carbs: 41 g., protein: 20 g., fiber: 6 g.

(quick meal) Tarragon Chicken Salad Boats

3 ounces cooked chicken breast (from rotisserie chicken), cubed

½ cup halved grapes

¼ cup thinly sliced celery

3 tablespoons 2 percent plain Greek yogurt

1 teaspoon honey

½ tablespoon freshly chopped tarragon

Salt and pepper to taste

2 romaine leaves

1 tablespoon slivered almonds

1. In a large bowl, combine the cooked chicken, sliced grapes, and celery.

2. In a small bowl, mix the yogurt, honey, and tarragon.

3. Toss the chicken with the dressing until the mixture is well combined, then season with salt and pepper.

4. Assemble the lettuce "boats" and top with the slivered almonds.

GLUTEN-FREE SUBSTITUTION: Naturally gluten-free!

VEGETARIAN SUBSTITUTION: Replace the chicken with ½ cup canned white beans.

SHORTCUT: Substitute ¾ teaspoon dried tarragon for fresh tarragon. Purchase prewashed and trimmed romaine leaves.

MONEY-SAVING TIP: What to do with extra tarragon? Place it in an airtight container and store it in the freezer for up to six months. Tarragon can be used to infuse oils or for future chicken recipes!

NUTRITION TIP: Romaine leaves make an excellent low-calorie nutrient-dense substitute for bread and crackers. Roll the romaine leaf for a wrap or use it as the base of an open-faced "sandwich."

Nutrition information: calories: 300, fat: 8 g., carbs: 26 g., protein: 33 g., fiber: 4 g.

Thai Turkey Lettuce Wraps

1 teaspoon unsalted butter

½ cup diced red bell pepper

4 ounces 93 percent lean ground turkey

1 garlic clove, minced

2 teaspoons soy sauce

½ tablespoon freshly grated ginger or 1 teaspoon ground ginger

¼ teaspoon cinnamon

2 teaspoons maple syrup

⅓ teaspoon crushed red pepper (optional)

½ cup shredded carrots

⅓ cup water

⅓ cup brown rice (from Sunday)

3 romaine lettuce leaves

2 tablespoons freshly chopped cilantro

1 tablespoon slivered almonds

1. Heat a frying pan over medium heat.

2. Add the butter and sauté the red bell peppers until they are soft (about 5 minutes); set the peppers aside.

3. In same frying pan, cook the turkey until it is browned, stirring frequently.

4. Add the garlic, soy sauce, ginger, cinnamon, maple syrup, crushed red pepper, and carrots and sauté the mixture over medium-high heat 3 minutes, stirring occasionally.

5. Reduce the heat to medium, add the water, and cook for another 5 minutes until most of the water evaporates.

6. Add the red bell peppers and rice to the pan and cook 1 minute, stirring until everything is well combined.

7. Place the turkey mixture evenly over romaine leaves and top each leaf with the fresh cilantro and slivered almonds.

GLUTEN-FREE SUBSTITUTION: Replace the soy sauce with gluten-free soy or tamari sauce.

VEGETARIAN SUBSTITUTION: Replace the turkey with ⅓ cup cooked lentils.

Nutrition information: calories: 390, fat: 10 g., carbs: 41 g., protein: 35 g., fiber: 8 g.

Monday SNACK

Veggies with Hummus and Fruit

5 3-inch carrot sticks
5 cherry tomatoes
2 tablespoons hummus
½ cup sliced strawberries

1. Wash and slice the veggies and fruit.

2. Dip the veggies in the hummus.

GLUTEN-FREE SUBSTITUTION: Naturally gluten-free!

Nutrition information: calories: 120, fat: 3.5 g., carbs: 21 g., protein: 4 g., fiber: 7 g.

The *Classic* Breakfast

1 chicken breakfast sausage
2 large eggs
1 teaspoon unsalted butter
½ sprouted whole-grain English muffin or 1 slice sprouted whole-grain bread
¾ cup blueberries

1. Heat a frying pan over medium heat.

2. Cook the sausage link according to the package directions; set the link aside.

3. Meanwhile, crack the eggs into a small bowl and, if scrambling them, whisk them with a fork.

4. Add the butter to the frying pan.

5. Once the butter evenly coats the pan, add the eggs.

6. Adjust the temperature to your preferred heat and either scramble the eggs, stirring them with a spatula till a desired doneness is reached, or fry the eggs sunny-side up, over easy, or to your liking.

7. Serve the eggs and sausage with the toast and blueberries.

GLUTEN-FREE SUBSTITUTION: Choose gluten-free bread.

VEGETARIAN SUBSTITUTION: Replace the chicken sausage with vegetarian sausage.

NUTRITION TIP: Did you know butter from pasture-raised cows contains higher amounts of conjugated linoleic acid (CLA)? Diets rich in CLA have been shown to help with weight management.[4]

Nutrition information: calories: 420, fat: 22 g., carbs: 34 g., protein: 25 g., fiber: 6 g.

Shrimp with Jicama and Mango Salad

3½ ounces shrimp, peeled and deveined
Salt and pepper to taste
½ tablespoon unsalted butter or coconut oil

SALAD
1½ cups cubed jicama
1 cup cubed mango
1 cup diced red bell pepper
¼ cup chopped red onion
2 tablespoons minced jalapeño (optional)
Juice of 2 limes
2 teaspoons extra-virgin olive oil
¼ cup freshly chopped cilantro

1. Heat a frying pan over medium heat.

2. Pat the shrimp dry with a paper towel and add a dash of salt and pepper.

3. Add the butter and shrimp to the pan and cook the shrimp until it is pink and opaque (2 to 3 minutes); set the shrimp aside.

4. For the salad, place the jicama, mango, red bell pepper, onion, and jalapeño in a bowl. Stir until the mixture is well combined.

5. Mix the lime juice and olive oil and pour the dressing over the salad.

6. Add the cilantro and toss the salad gently. Reserve half the salad for tomorrow's snack.

7. Serve the remaining salad with the shrimp.

GLUTEN-FREE SUBSTITUTION: Naturally gluten-free!

VEGETARIAN SUBSTITUTION: Replace the shrimp with ½ cup canned black beans.

INGREDIENT SUBSTITUTION: If fresh mango is not available, use fresh pineapple.

SHORTCUT: Buy peeled and deveined shrimp from the fish counter.

GROCERY GUIDE: Get to know your fishmonger! Fishmongers have a wealth of information on preparing fish and are sure to help with perfect portions.

Nutrition information: calories: 280, fat: 12 g., carbs: 29 g., protein: 16 g., fiber: 8 g.

Tuesday DINNER

quick meal Sundried Tomato, Feta, and Spinach Chicken Salad

2 cups baby spinach

4 ounces cooked chicken breast (from rotisserie chicken), chopped

⅓ cup cooked and chilled brown rice (from Sunday)

2 tablespoons chopped sundried tomatoes packed in oil

1 tablespoon balsamic vinegar

¾ ounce feta cheese

2 fresh basil leaves, chopped

1. In a medium bowl, place the spinach, chicken, rice, and sundried tomatoes.

2. Add the vinegar and feta cheese and toss gently.

3. Top the salad with fresh basil.

GLUTEN-FREE SUBSTITUTION: Naturally gluten-free!

VEGETARIAN SUBSTITUTION: Replace the chicken with ½ cup canned white beans.

GROCERY GUIDE: Look for sundried tomatoes stored in extra-virgin olive oil. A little goes a long way; sundried tomatoes are packed with flavor and the additional healthy monounsaturated fat helps you better absorb vitamins A and K from the spinach.

NUTRITION TIP: Balsamic vinegar gives your salads an excellent "tang" while promoting satiety. Research shows that vinegar can act as an appetite suppressant, making it easier to stick to your meal plan!

Nutrition information: calories: 370, fat: 11 g., carbs: 30 g., protein: 39 g., fiber: 4 g.

Dill Dip with Pita "Chips" and Veggies

½ sprouted whole-grain pita
¼ cup 2 percent plain Greek yogurt
1 teaspoon lemon juice
1 teaspoon freshly chopped dill
⅓ teaspoon garlic powder, or to taste
½ small yellow bell pepper, sliced
½ cucumber, sliced into rounds

1. Toast the ½ pita and slice it into 4 wedges.

2. In a small bowl, mix the Greek yogurt, lemon juice, dill, and garlic powder until the dip is well combined.

3. Enjoy the dip with the yellow bell pepper slices, cucumber, and pita "chips."

GLUTEN-FREE SUBSTITUTION: Omit the pita "chips" and enjoy ½ cup seedless grapes.

Nutrition information: calories: 130, fat: 2 g., carbs: 21 g., protein: 9 g., fiber: 4 g.

Smoked Salmon Flatbread

1 sprouted whole-grain tortilla
2 tablespoons whipped cream cheese
1 tomato, sliced
⅓ red onion, thinly sliced (optional)
3 ounces wild smoked salmon
1 teaspoon freshly chopped dill
½ apple, sliced

1. Toast the tortilla in the oven until it is golden brown.

2. Spread the cream cheese evenly over the tortilla.

3. Arrange the tomatoes and onion across the tortilla.

4. Place the smoked salmon on top and finish with fresh dill.

5. Enjoy with the apple slices.

GLUTEN-FREE SUBSTITUTION: Choose a sprouted brown-rice tortilla.

VEGETARIAN SUBSTITUTION: Replace the salmon with ½ cup canned garbanzo beans, rinsed. Swap out the cream cheese for 1½ ounces goat cheese.

NUTRITION TIP: Did you know that dill is not only a flavorful herb but also helpful in aiding healthy digestion?

Nutrition information: calories: 350, fat: 14 g., carbs: 36 g., protein: 21 g., fiber: 6 g.

quick meal Grab-and-Go Lunch

This lunch will take you back to your childhood. Remember ants on a log? This one doesn't have raisins but does have some extra protein to keep you full!

1½ tablespoons almond butter
1½ stalks celery, cut into 3-inch sticks
3 ounces turkey luncheon meat
½ cup grapes

1. Spread the almond butter evenly over the celery sticks, or use the sticks to dip.
2. Enjoy with sliced turkey and grapes.

GLUTEN-FREE SUBSTITUTION: Naturally gluten-free!

VEGETARIAN SUBSTITUTION: Replace the turkey with ½ cup edamame.

QUICK SWAP: On the road? Starbucks sells a Protein Bistro Box that could replace this meal; just reserve the apples and peanut butter as your snack.

NUTRITION TIP: Almond butter has more heart-friendly monounsaturated fats and is higher in omega-3s (alpha-linolenic acid) than peanut butter.

Nutrition information: calories: 300, fat: 15 g., carbs: 21 g., protein: 27 g., fiber: 5 g.

REVVED-Up Soup

Makes 2 3-cup servings

8 ounces 93 percent lean ground turkey
½ tablespoon unsalted butter
1 cup chopped carrot
½ cup chopped celery
¼ cup chopped red onion
2 garlic cloves, minced
1½ cups canned fire-roasted tomatoes
1½ cups cubed frozen butternut squash
1 cup frozen green beans
½ teaspoon dried basil
½ teaspoon dried oregano
1 teaspoon freshly chopped parsley
1 teaspoon whole fennel seed
½ teaspoon salt
½ cup canned white beans, rinsed
2 cups *REVVED* Chicken Bone Broth or chicken stock
1 tablespoon shredded Parmesan cheese (for dinner portion only)

1. Heat a medium-size saucepan over medium heat.

2. Brown the turkey and set it aside in a separate bowl.

3. Return the pan to the burner and add the butter, followed by the carrots and celery.

4. Sauté the carrots and celery until they are soft (about 5 minutes).

5. Add the onion and cook the mixture an additional 3 minutes, stirring frequently.

6. Incorporate the garlic and cook until it is fragrant.

7. Add the tomatoes, squash, green beans, basil, oregano, parsley, fennel, and salt. Cook the mixture 2 minutes until the spices become fragrant.

8. Add the turkey, white beans, and chicken broth.

9. Bring the soup to a low boil, then reduce the heat and simmer it for 10 minutes.

10. Serve half the soup with the Parmesan cheese. (Store the remaining soup in an airtight glass container in the refrigerator for tomorrow's lunch.)

GLUTEN-FREE SUBSTITUTION: Naturally gluten-free!

VEGETARIAN SUBSTITUTION: Replace the turkey with ¼ cup lentils (uncooked) and swap out the chicken broth for vegetarian broth. Top the soup with 2 tablespoons cheese. Increase the broth to 20 ounces

NUTRITION TIP: Fennel seed adds a unique, deep flavor to this soup. It also has been shown to aid in digestion and help reduce bloating.

Nutrition information: calories: 400, fat: 8 g., carbs: 46 g., protein: 40 g., fiber: 13 g.

Wednesday SNACK

Jicama and Mango Salad

Half of the batch of Jicama and Mango Salad made at lunch yesterday is stored in the refrigerator for today's snack.

GLUTEN-FREE SUBSTITUTION: Naturally gluten-free!

Nutrition information: calories: 160, fat: 5 g., carbs: 29 g., protein: 2 g., fiber: 8 g.

(quick meal) Mediterranean Breakfast Sandwich and Fruit

Even if you are rushing out the door in the morning, you can assemble this sandwich in minutes, and it's a great commuter-friendly breakfast to get you *REVVED* for the day.

- 1 sprouted whole-grain English muffin
- 2 ounces turkey luncheon meat
- 2 slices tomato
- ½ cup baby spinach
- 2 leaves fresh basil
- 1 ounce feta cheese or 2 tablespoons whipped cream cheese
- 3 olives, sliced
- ½ cup blueberries

1. Assemble the English muffin, turkey, tomato, spinach, basil, cheese, and olives into a sandwich and serve it with the blueberries.

2. If time permits, toast the English muffin.

GLUTEN-FREE SUBSTITUTION: Swap out the English muffin for a gluten-free sprouted brown-rice tortilla.

VEGETARIAN SUBSTITUTION: Replace the turkey with 1 hard-boiled egg and 1 egg white, crumbled.

NUTRITION TIP: Baby spinach is a nutrition powerhouse. It is packed with fiber, folate, and vitamins A and K. Pick up a bag of prewashed baby spinach and add it to sandwiches, omelets, or smoothies. It's a wonderful way to add nutrients and fiber to any meal!

Nutrition information: calories: 380, fat: 10 g., carbs: 46 g., protein: 27 g., fiber: 9 g.

Thursday LUNCH

(quick meal) *REVVED*-Up Soup

Half of the batch of *REVVED*-Up Soup made for yesterday's dinner is in the refrigerator for today's lunch.

Nutrition information: calories: 370, fat: 5 g., carbs: 46 g., protein: 37 g., fiber: 13 g.

Thursday DINNER

(quick meal) Parmesan Tilapia with Sundried Tomatoes and Green Beans Almondine

6 ounces tilapia or cod

2 tablespoons 2 percent plain Greek yogurt

⅓ teaspoon garlic powder

2 tablespoons shredded Parmesan cheese

Salt and pepper to taste

1 cup frozen green beans

Juice of ½ lemon

1 tablespoon slivered almonds

2 tablespoons chopped sundried tomatoes packed in oil

2 leaves fresh basil, chopped (optional)

1. Turn the oven on to broil; adjust the rack so it is about 6 inches from the broiler.

2. Line a baking sheet with foil.

3. Place the tilapia in the center of the baking sheet.

4. Spread the yogurt evenly over the fish. Top the fish with garlic powder and cheese, and season with salt and pepper.

5. Broil the fish 3 to 5 minutes (depending on the thickness), being careful not to overcook it.

6. Meanwhile, steam the green beans either on the stovetop or in the microwave.

7. Add the lemon juice and almonds to the green beans and toss them gently. Add salt and pepper to taste.

8. Top the fish with the sundried tomatoes and fresh basil.

GLUTEN-FREE SUBSTITUTION: Naturally gluten-free!

VEGETARIAN SUBSTITUTION: Replace the fish with a vegetarian patty, such as a Sunshine Burger.

NUTRITION TIP: Stovetop or microwave? In an *ideal* world, we'd have plenty of time to prepare meals the old-fashioned way. Unfortunately, schedules don't always permit lengthy food preparation. If you are short on time, don't be afraid to resort to the microwave to steam your veggies. Research shows that microwaving may help preserve some of the heat-sensitive nutrients.[5] But if you have the time, grab that steaming basket. Just don't boil green beans in water, because the water-soluble vitamins leach into the water, leaving you with tasteless, nutrient-deficient mush!

Nutrition information: calories: 340, fat: 14 g., carbs: 11 g., protein: 46 g., fiber: 3 g.

Spiced Garbanzo Bites

Makes 2 ⅓-cup servings

⅓ cup canned garbanzo beans, rinsed
1 teaspoon unsalted butter, melted, or coconut oil
2 teaspoons maple syrup
½ teaspoon pumpkin pie spice
Dash of salt (optional)

1. Preheat the oven to 350°F.

2. Line a baking sheet with parchment paper.

3. Place the rinsed garbanzo beans on paper towels and pat them dry. Transfer the beans to the baking sheet and discard the paper towels.

4. Bake the beans for 35 minutes, stirring them after 20 minutes.

5. In a small bowl, toss the beans with the melted butter, maple syrup, pumpkin pie spice, and dash of salt.

6. Return the beans to the parchment-lined baking sheet and bake them an additional 5 minutes.

7. Let them cool. Enjoy half of them for your snack, and store the remainder for tomorrow's snack. These will keep in an airtight container for up to three days.

GLUTEN-FREE SUBSTITUTION: Naturally gluten-free!

Nutrition information (per serving): calories: 110, fat: 2.5 g., carbs: 19 g., protein: 4 g., fiber: 4 g.

Chorizo Breakfast Burrito and Melon

Makes 2 servings

2½ ounces chorizo
2 teaspoons unsalted butter
½ cup chopped red bell peppers
¼ cup chopped red onion
2 eggs
2 egg whites
2 sprouted whole-grain tortillas
1 tablespoon freshly chopped cilantro
½ cup cubed cantaloupe

1. Heat a frying pan over medium heat.

2. Cook the chorizo until it is browned, stirring it occasionally, and set it aside in a small bowl.

3. Add the butter to the pan and sauté the peppers and onions until they are soft.

4. Combine the eggs and egg whites in a bowl, whisk them with a fork, and add them to the pan.

5. Using a spatula, scramble the eggs to a desired doneness.

6. Return the chorizo to the pan and stir the mixture until it is well incorporated.

7. Place half the mixture on each tortilla, add the cilantro, and roll each up into a burrito. Serve one with melon.

8. Once cooled, store the second burrito in an airtight container or plastic wrap in the freezer for Week 3.

GLUTEN-FREE SUBSTITUTION: Choose a sprouted brown-rice tortilla.

VEGETARIAN SUBSTITUTION: Replace the chorizo with 1 additional whole egg. For extra spice, add ⅓ teaspoon crushed red pepper.

INGREDIENT SUBSTITUTION: Not a chorizo fan? Swap out the chorizo for any flavored sausage.

QUANTITY TIP: One ounce of chorizo is about one-third to one-quarter of a medium sausage link. Although a small amount of meat, it sure does pack a ton of flavor. When making this recipe, consider quadrupling the batch. These burritos freeze well and can be the perfect grab-and-go breakfast when in a hurry. Or share them with the rest of the family—they are sure to be a huge hit!

NUTRITION TIP: Cantaloupe is an excellent source of beta-carotene, an antioxidant shown to promote healthy skin, hair, and aging.

Nutrition information: calories: 410, fat: 22 g., carbs: 34 g., protein: 20 g., fiber: 5 g.

Friday LUNCH

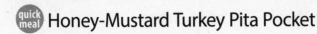 Honey-Mustard Turkey Pita Pocket

2 ounces turkey luncheon meat, chopped

¼ cup shredded carrots

1 cup chopped romaine lettuce

3 cherry tomatoes, halved

⅓ cup 2 percent plain Greek yogurt

½ tablespoon honey

2 teaspoons Dijon mustard

1 tablespoon freshly chopped parsley (optional)

Dash of salt and pepper

1 sprouted whole-grain pita

1. In a large bowl, combine the turkey, carrots, lettuce, and tomatoes.

2. In a small bowl, mix yogurt, honey, mustard, parsley, salt, and pepper.

3. Toss the turkey mixture with the dressing until everything is well combined.

4. Fill the pita and enjoy.

GLUTEN-FREE SUBSTITUTION: Choose a gluten-free pita bread or brown-rice tortilla.

VEGETARIAN SUBSTITUTION: Swap ½ cup canned garbanzo beans for the turkey.

GROCERY GUIDE: Pick a pita that is made with 100 percent whole grains. Check the ingredient list. If you see the word "enriched," select a different brand.

NUTRITION TIP: Sprinkle parsley on your favorite salads and soups. Not only will it add delicious flavor and depth but it will also aid in digestion and help with bloating.

Nutrition information: calories: 260, fat: 3 g., carbs: 40 g., protein: 22 g., fiber: 5 g.

Savory Maple-Glazed Salmon with Roasted Rosemary Butternut Squash and Steamed Broccoli

1 cup cubed butternut squash
1 tablespoon butter
1½ teaspoons dried rosemary
4 ounces wild salmon
1 teaspoon chili powder
Dash of salt and pepper, or to taste
2 teaspoons maple syrup
1 cup frozen broccoli, steamed

1. Preheat the oven to 400°F.

2. Toss the butternut squash with 2 teaspoons of the butter, melted, and the rosemary and place the squash on a baking sheet.

3. Roast the pieces for 10 minutes; flip them with a spatula, and roast them an additional 10 minutes or until they are golden brown.

4. While the butternut squash cooks, heat a frying pan over medium heat.

5. Add the remaining 1 teaspoon of butter to the pan.

6. Season the salmon with the chili powder, salt, and pepper.

7. Cook the salmon skin side down for 2 minutes, flip it up on its side for 30 seconds, repeat the same on the other side, and then finish cooking it skin side down. Add the maple syrup during the last 2 minutes of cooking, using a spoon to catch the syrup and coat the fish evenly.

8. Cook the salmon until its internal temperature reaches 145°F, or to the desired doneness.

9. Serve the fish with the steamed broccoli and butternut squash.

GLUTEN-FREE SUBSTITUTION: Naturally gluten-free!

VEGETARIAN SUBSTITUTION: Replace the salmon with 8 ounces extra-firm tofu.

GROCERY GUIDE: When in season, look for precut butternut squash in your produce section rather than the frozen section for optimal texture. Remember to adjust the cooking time accordingly, depending on the size of the butternut cubes.

> **NUTRITION TIP:** The omega-3 fatty acids DHA and EPA can degrade during the cooking process. To help preserve these healthy fats, make sure to incorporate rosemary in the meal. Research has shown that rosemary helps prevent the oxidation of heat-sensitive omega-3s.[6]

Nutrition information: calories: 420, fat: 19 g., carbs: 36 g., protein: 30 g., fiber: 9 g.

Friday SNACK

Spiced Garbanzo Bites

Half of the batch of Spiced Garbanzo Bites made for yesterday's snack is stored in an airtight container for today's snack.

Nutrition information: calories: 110, fat: 2.5 g., carbs: 19 g., protein: 4 g., fiber: 4 g.

(quick meal) Chocolate-Banana Protein Shake

- 1 scoop whey protein powder
- 1 cup 2 percent milk
- ½ banana
- 1 tablespoon unsweetened cocoa powder
- 1 tablespoon almond butter
- 1 cup baby spinach
- 1 cup ice (optional)

Place all the ingredients in a blender and blend the mixture until it's smooth.

GLUTEN-FREE SUBSTITUTION: Naturally gluten-free, but double-check the label on your protein powder.

NUTRITION TIP: Dark cocoa is rich in flavonoids and antioxidants shown to boost heart health, improve insulin sensitivity, and promote healthy aging.[7]

Nutrition information: calories: 380, fat: 15 g., carbs: 37 g., protein: 34 g., fiber: 6 g.

Mediterranean Salad

½ cup canned garbanzo beans, rinsed
3 olives, pitted and chopped
1 tomato, chopped
½ cucumber, chopped
2 tablespoons chopped red onion
¾ ounces feta cheese, crumbled
1 tablespoon lemon juice
1 teaspoon extra-virgin olive oil
2 tablespoons freshly chopped parsley
2 fresh basil leaves, torn into small pieces (optional)
Salt and pepper (optional)
½ cup seedless grapes, rinsed

1. In a medium bowl, combine the beans, olives, tomato, cucumber, onion, and cheese.

2. Add the lemon juice, olive oil, parsley, basil, and a dash of salt and pepper. Toss the mixture gently.

3. Enjoy the salad with a side of grapes.

GLUTEN-FREE SUBSTITUTION: Naturally gluten-free!

NUTRITION TIP: Although soaking and cooking your own beans is the optimal choice (less salt and fewer gut irritants), canned beans are incredibly convenient. Make sure to rinse canned beans well to reduce their sodium content up to 40 percent.

NUTRITION TIP: A little goes a long way with feta cheese! Just a small amount adds richness and flavor to any dish. This soft cheese has one-third fewer calories and fat compared to hard cheeses such as cheddar.

Nutrition information: calories: 350, fat: 13 g., carbs: 48 g., protein: 13 g., fiber: 6 g.

Cumin-Spiced Flank Steak with Roasted Sweet Potato and Sautéed Veggies

With this recipe, the most labor-intensive one of the bunch, you will do one prep for two meals. For optimal flavor, marinate the steak for a minimum of 2 hours.

1 9-ounce flank steak

MARINADE
¼ cup extra-virgin olive oil
1 tablespoon balsamic vinegar
Juice of 1 lime
¼ cup freshly chopped cilantro
2 tablespoons honey
1 teaspoon cumin
Salt and pepper to taste

VEGGIES
1 large sweet potato
2 teaspoons butter
½ yellow onion, sliced
2 red bell peppers, sliced
2 teaspoons balsamic vinegar

1. Place the steak in a shallow glass dish. Mix all the marinade ingredients and pour it over the steak. Cover the dish and place it in the refrigerator for at least 2 hours.

2. Preheat the oven to 400°F.

3. Place the sweet potato on a baking sheet and bake it for 45 minutes or until it is tender.

4. Discard the marinade and pat the steak dry with a paper towel. Let it rest for 10 minutes.

5. Heat a frying pan over medium heat.

6. Add the butter, let it melt, and then add the onion and a dash of salt.

7. Lower the heat to medium-low and cook the onions for 10 minutes, stirring occasionally.

8. Increase the heat to medium, add the sliced peppers, and cook them for 5 to 10 minutes, stirring frequently.

9. Add the balsamic vinegar to the pepper and onion mixture and cook an additional minute, stirring occasionally.

10. Preheat a grill to medium-high.

11. Grill the steak for 4 minutes on each side or until it reaches a desired doneness. (An internal reading of 145°F will produce a medium steak after resting 10 minutes.)

12. Remove the steak from the grill and let it rest at least 10 minutes. Slice the steak against the grain into thin strips.

13. Serve half of the steak strips, half of the pepper and onion mixture, and half of the sweet potato. (Save the remaining steak, pepper and onion mixture, and sweet potato for tomorrow's lunch.)

GLUTEN-FREE SUBSTITUTION: Naturally gluten-free!

VEGETARIAN SUBSTITUTION: Replace the steak with 6 ounces extra-firm tofu. Marinate as instructed. Discard the marinade, and pat the tofu dry with a paper towel. For a crispy texture, make sure to drain the excess liquid from the tofu (placing extra paper towels under the tofu and a heavy kitchen plate on top of the tofu for 10 minutes should do the trick). Sauté the tofu in a separate pan over medium-high heat. Serve with ⅓ cup canned black beans.

> **NUTRITION TIP:** Why is it important to choose 100 percent grass-fed and finished meats? One hundred percent grass-fed meats have been shown to have higher levels of vitamins A and E and conjugated linoleic acid (CLA), and CLA has been shown to help with weight management. Some meats labeled grass-fed are not 100 percent grass-fed; the cattle are sent to feeding lots for their last month or two. During this time, the CLA content can decrease by 30 to 40 percent.[8] Ask your butcher if your meat is 100 percent grass-fed *and* finished!

Nutrition information: calories: 390, fat: 15 g., carbs: 28 g., protein: 33 g., fiber: 5 g.

Cantaloupe and Greek Yogurt

⅓ cup 2 percent plain Greek yogurt
Dash of cinnamon (optional)
1 cup cubed cantaloupe

Sprinkle the cinnamon on the yogurt and enjoy with the melon.

GLUTEN-FREE SUBSTITUTION: Naturally gluten-free!

Nutrition information: calories: 110, fat: 2 g., carbs: 16 g., protein: 8 g., fiber: 1 g.

Sunday BREAKFAST

Turkey and Sweet Potato Hash

1½ teaspoons coconut oil
⅓ cup diced sweet potato
3 tablespoons chopped yellow onion
3 ounces 93 percent lean ground turkey
1 teaspoon maple syrup
½ teaspoon pumpkin pie spice or cinnamon
½ cup apple, peeled and chopped
Salt and pepper to taste
¼ cup water

1. Heat a skillet over medium heat.

2. Add 1 teaspoon of the coconut oil and the sweet potato, and sauté the sweet potato until it is golden brown; set it aside.

3. Add the remaining ½ teaspoon coconut oil and the onion to the pan and sauté the onion until it is soft; set it aside.

4. Add the turkey to the pan and cook it until it is browned.

5. Return the sweet potato and onions to the pan. Add the maple syrup, pumpkin pie spice, apples (store the remaining apple for Monday's lunch), salt, and pepper, and stir the hash until it is well combined.

6. Add the water and cook the mixture until the water evaporates, stirring frequently (about 5 minutes).

GLUTEN-FREE SUBSTITUTION: Naturally gluten-free!

VEGETARIAN SUBSTITUTION: Replace the turkey with vegetarian ground "turkey."

NUTRITION TIP: Creating a breakfast hash is a great way to start your morning with a solid serving of lean protein and veggies. As an extra bonus, it is a great way to use leftover meat and veggies!

STORAGE TIP: Store the remaining apple, unpeeled and unchopped, in the fridge, flesh side down on a small plate, or if you're on the go, place it in an airtight container with a touch of lemon juice to prevent browning.

Nutrition information: calories: 360, fat: 9 g., carbs: 43 g., protein: 31 g., fiber: 4 g.

Sunday LUNCH

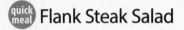 Flank Steak Salad

You will be using the other half of the steak, onion and pepper mixture, and sweet potato you prepared for last night's dinner.

    2 cups chopped romaine lettuce
    Remaining flank steak (about 3½ ounces cooked)
    Remaining sweet potato, chopped
    Remaining pepper and onion mixture
    4 cherry tomatoes, halved
    Juice of ½ lime
    1 teaspoon extra-virgin olive oil

1. Place the lettuce in a medium bowl.

2. Add the steak, sweet potato, pepper and onion mixture, and cherry tomatoes.

3. Add the lime juice and olive oil, and toss gently.

GLUTEN-FREE SUBSTITUTION: Naturally gluten-free!

VEGETARIAN SUBSTITUTION: Replace the flank steak with ½ cup canned black beans.

GROCERY GUIDE: Flank steak shrinks while cooking, leaving about 80 percent of its original weight. Keep this in mind when grocery shopping and ordering at restaurants.

Nutrition information: calories: 360, fat: 16 g., carbs: 33 g., protein: 23 g., fiber: 8 g.

Sunday DINNER

quick meal Spicy Southwest Chicken Sandwich with Veggies

½ sprouted whole-grain English muffin or 1 slice sprouted whole-grain bread

1 romaine leaf, torn into 2 or 3 pieces

3 ounces chicken breast (from rotisserie chicken)

½ large yellow bell pepper, sliced

⅓ cucumber, sliced into rounds

SPICY SAUCE

¾ cup 2 percent plain Greek yogurt

½ small canned chipotle pepper, minced (more if you like it extra spicy)

½ teaspoon adobo sauce

½ teaspoon chili powder

½ teaspoon cumin

1 tablespoon honey

Juice of 1 lime

½ tablespoon apple cider vinegar

2 tablespoons freshly chopped cilantro

1. In a small bowl, mix the ingredients for the Spicy Sauce. (Reserve ⅓ cup for tomorrow's snack.)

2. If necessary, slice the chicken to fit on the bread.

3. Spread 1 to 2 tablespoons of sauce on the bread; top the sauce with the romaine and then the chicken.

4. Enjoy this open-faced sandwich with a side of bell peppers, cucumber rounds, and remaining sauce for dipping.

GLUTEN-FREE SUBSTITUTION: Swap the bread for gluten-free bread or a brown-rice tortilla.

VEGETARIAN SUBSTITUTION: Replace the chicken with a vegetarian patty, such as a Sunshine Burger.

GROCERY GUIDE: Look for chipotle peppers in adobo sauce in the Mexican section of your grocery store. Freeze leftover chipotle peppers and adobo sauce in an ice cube tray and store the cubes in the freezer for up to three months.

Nutrition information: calories: 360, fat: 6 g., carbs: 40 g., protein: 39 g., fiber: 6 g.

Sunday SNACK

Guacamole and Veggies

8 3-inch carrot sticks or 1 bell pepper, sliced
1 mini container guacamole (100-calories)

Dip the veggies in the guacamole and enjoy!

GROCERY GUIDE: Check out the produce section for 100-calorie packs of guacamole. These make the perfect heart-healthy snack. Don't worry about waste; these convenient snacks can be stored in the freezer for several months.

GLUTEN-FREE SUBSTITUTION: Naturally gluten-free!

Nutrition information: calories: 130, fat: 8 g., carbs: 11 g., protein: 3 g., fiber: 6 g.

Monday BREAKFAST

quick meal Triple-B Protein Shake

1 cup 2 percent milk
1 scoop whey protein powder
½ banana
½ cup frozen blueberries
¾ cup frozen broccoli
10 almonds

1. Place the milk, protein powder, banana, blueberries, and broccoli in a blender and blend the mixture until it is smooth.

2. Enjoy the shake with a small handful of almonds (about 10).

GLUTEN-FREE SUBSTITUTION: Naturally gluten-free!

INGREDIENT SUBSTITUTION: Not a fan of broccoli? Feel free to replace it with 1 cup baby spinach. Adding veggies to your smoothie is a surefire way to get your metabolism *REVVED* up for the day.

Nutrition information: calories: 400, fat: 13 g., carbs: 47 g., protein: 34 g., fiber: 8 g.

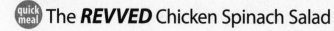 The *REVVED* Chicken Spinach Salad

3 ounces cooked chicken breast (from rotisserie chicken), shredded

2 cups baby spinach

5 cherry tomatoes, halved

¼ cup shredded carrots

½ apple, chopped (include any remaining from Sunday's breakfast)

⅓ cup chopped cucumber

DRESSING

½ teaspoon balsamic vinegar

½ teaspoon honey

½ teaspoon Dijon mustard

Dash of cumin

1 tablespoon extra-virgin olive oil

½ tablespoon water

1. Place the chicken, spinach, tomatoes, carrots, apple, and cucumber in a medium bowl.

2. In a small bowl, mix well all the dressing ingredients with a fork.

3. Add the dressing to the salad and toss gently.

GLUTEN-FREE SUBSTITUTION: Naturally gluten-free!

VEGETARIAN SUBSTITUTION: Replace the chicken with 2 hard-boiled eggs and 1 hard-boiled egg white.

SHORTCUT: *Mise en place* means "putting in place." In the culinary world *mise en place* refers to preparing ingredients in advance and storing them for later use. To assemble meals quickly, set aside one prep day per week to chop vegetables and herbs. Store them in airtight glass containers in the fridge and use them as needed.

GROCERY GUIDE: Look for 100 percent extra-virgin olive oil in a dark glass bottle. Olive oil is subject to oxidation, so exposure to light and heat can destroy this healthy fat.

NUTRITION TIP: Tomatoes are an excellent source of lycopene, a potent antioxidant shown to reduce the risk of certain cancers and promote healthy aging.

Nutrition information: calories: 300, fat: 10 g., carbs: 27 g., protein: 28 g., fiber: 7 g.

Maple-Mustard Pork Loin with Roasted Butternut Squash Puree

For optimal flavor, marinate the pork for at least 2 hours.

4 ounces boneless pork loin
2½ teaspoons maple syrup
½ teaspoon soy sauce
1½ teaspoons Dijon mustard
1 teaspoon extra-virgin olive oil
1 cup cubed frozen butternut squash
Cooking spray
Salt and pepper
1 tablespoon 2 percent milk
½ teaspoon unsalted butter
5 cherry tomatoes
1 cup frozen broccoli, steamed

1. Marinate the pork in an airtight container in 1½ teaspoons of the maple syrup, the soy sauce, the Dijon mustard, and the olive oil in the refrigerator for 2 hours.

2. Preheat the oven to 350°F.

3. Line a baking sheet with foil or parchment paper.

4. Place the squash on the baking sheet, lightly coat the pieces with cooking spray, and season them with salt and pepper.

5. Bake the squash on an upper rack for 10 minutes, rotate them on the baking sheet, and continue cooking them until they are golden brown.

6. Meanwhile, transfer the pork and the marinade to an oven-safe dish. Bake it for 15 minutes or until the meat's internal temperature reaches 145°F. Let it rest 10 minutes.

7. While the pork rests, place the butternut squash in a food processor with the remaining 1 teaspoon maple syrup, the milk, and the butter. Puree the mixture until it is smooth.

8. Place the cherry tomatoes in a baking pan and bake them for 5 to 10 minutes, until they are soft.

9. Serve the pork with the squash, steamed broccoli, and roasted tomatoes.

GLUTEN-FREE SUBSTITUTION: Use gluten-free soy or tamari sauce.

VEGETARIAN SUBSTITUTION: Replace the pork with 8 ounces extra-firm tofu. Cut the tofu into bite-size cubes and cook them on the stovetop until they are golden brown.

INGREDIENT SUBSTITUTION: Not a pork fan? Replace it with skinless chicken or turkey breast.

Nutrition information: calories: 390, fat: 15 g., carbs: 40 g., protein: 28 g., fiber: 7 g.

Plan ahead! Remember to make more *REVVED* Chicken Bone Broth (see recipe on p. 122) for tomorrow's dinner.

Monday SNACK

Spicy Dipping Sauce and Veggies

You will have ⅓ cup Spicy Sauce in the refrigerator from last night's dinner.

½ cup sliced yellow bell pepper (about 5 strips)
5 3-inch carrot sticks
⅓ cup Spicy Sauce

Dip the veggies in the Spicy Sauce and enjoy!

GLUTEN-FREE SUBSTITUTION: Naturally gluten-free!

INGREDIENT SUBSTITUTION: Feel free to utilize any nonstarchy vegetable with this dip, such as broccoli, celery, cucumber, carrots, zucchini, or cauliflower. Aim for about a 1-cup serving.

Nutrition information: calories: 110, fat: 1.5 g., carbs: 19 g., protein: 7 g., fiber: 2 g.

The *REVVED* Omelet

This omelet is so packed full of veggies that it is best served "open-faced."

- ½ tablespoon unsalted butter
- 2 large eggs
- 2 egg whites
- 1 ounce goat cheese
- ½ cup baby spinach
- ⅓ cup diced zucchini
- ½ tomato, chopped
- 1 clementine or small piece of other fruit

1. Heat a frying pan over medium heat.

2. Whisk the eggs and egg whites in a small bowl.

3. Add the butter to the pan, let it melt, and then add the eggs. Once the eggs begin to firm around the edges, add the cheese, spinach, zucchini, and tomato.

4. Cover the pan with a lid and cook the omelet 3 to 4 minutes or until it reaches a desired doneness.

5. Transfer it to a plate and enjoy it with a clementine.

GLUTEN-FREE SUBSTITUTION: Naturally gluten-free!

NUTRITION TIP: Winter fruit options can be limited in certain areas. Avoid dried fruits, as they tend to be easy to overconsume and are more concentrated in sugar, causing a more rapid increase in blood-glucose levels. Check out your grocer's freezer section for a variety of low-glycemic fruits, such as blueberries, raspberries, and cherries.

Nutrition information: calories: 360, fat: 22 g., carbs: 16 g., protein: 26 g., fiber: 4 g.

Tuesday LUNCH

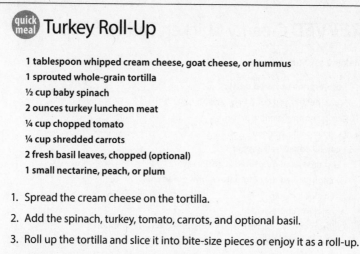 Turkey Roll-Up

1 tablespoon whipped cream cheese, goat cheese, or hummus
1 sprouted whole-grain tortilla
½ cup baby spinach
2 ounces turkey luncheon meat
¼ cup chopped tomato
¼ cup shredded carrots
2 fresh basil leaves, chopped (optional)
1 small nectarine, peach, or plum

1. Spread the cream cheese on the tortilla.

2. Add the spinach, turkey, tomato, carrots, and optional basil.

3. Roll up the tortilla and slice it into bite-size pieces or enjoy it as a roll-up.

4. Serve the roll-up with a piece of fruit.

GLUTEN-FREE SUBSTITUTION: Replace the whole-grain tortilla with a gluten-free brown-rice tortilla.

VEGETARIAN SUBSTITUTION: Replace the turkey with ½ cup sliced mushrooms and increase the amount of cream cheese to 2 tablespoons.

Nutrition information: calories: 300, fat: 8 g., carbs: 41 g., protein: 21 g., fiber: 7 g.

REVVED Creamy Chicken Tortilla Soup

Makes 2 servings

1 tablespoon unsalted butter

¾ cup peeled and cubed sweet potato

⅓ cup chopped yellow onion

2 cloves garlic, minced

1 cup diced red bell pepper

1 cup sliced and quartered zucchini

1½ cups canned diced tomatoes with green chilis

½ teaspoon cumin

½ teaspoon chili powder

7 ounces cooked chicken (from rotisserie chicken), chopped

2 cups *REVVED* Chicken Bone Broth

½ teaspoon salt

½ corn tortilla (for dinner serving *only*)

½ cup 2 percent plain Greek yogurt

¼ cup freshly chopped cilantro

1. Heat a medium saucepan over medium heat.

2. Add the butter and sweet potato and cook the sweet potato for 5 minutes, stirring it occasionally.

3. Add the onion and cook, stirring gently, until the onion is soft (about 3 minutes).

4. Add the garlic and stir until it is fragrant.

5. Add the red bell peppers, zucchini, tomatoes, cumin, and chili powder. Stir the mixture until it is well combined.

6. Add the chicken, broth, and salt.

7. Bring the soup to a gentle boil, reduce the heat, and simmer it for at least 10 minutes.

8. While the soup simmers, turn on the broiler.

9. Place the corn tortilla on a baking sheet coated with a touch of cooking spray.

10. Broil the tortilla until it is crispy; set it aside.

11. Remove the soup from the heat, add the yogurt, and stir the soup gently.

12. Cut or break the tortilla into bite-size pieces.

13. Serve half of the soup with all the cilantro and all the tortilla pieces.

14. Reserve the remaining soup for tomorrow's lunch.

GLUTEN-FREE SUBSTITUTION: Naturally gluten-free!

VEGETARIAN SUBSTITUTION: Replace the chicken with 1 cup canned white beans and the chicken broth with vegetable broth.

> **NUTRITION TIP:** Avoid canned soups and prepared soups from your local deli. They tend to be skimpy on the veggies and have an overabundance of cream. Instead, set aside 30 minutes per week to make a delicious and nutritious soup. Aim for at least 1 cup of vegetables per serving and choose a lean source of protein, such as chicken or turkey.

Nutrition information: calories: 420, fat: 13 g., carbs: 40 g., protein: 41 g., fiber: 10 g.

Cheesy Garlic Kale Chips

2 cups stemmed and chopped kale, cut into generous "chip"-size pieces
1 teaspoon extra-virgin olive oil
1½ tablespoons nutritional yeast flakes
¼ teaspoon onion powder
¼ teaspoon garlic powder
Salt and pepper to taste

1. Preheat the oven to 350°F.

2. Pat the kale dry to remove any moisture and place the pieces in a medium bowl.

3. Add the olive oil and toss to evenly coat the kale.

4. Add the nutritional yeast, onion powder, garlic powder, salt and pepper, and toss again.

5. Distribute the kale evenly on a baking sheet, making sure the pieces are not touching each other.

6. Bake the kale 10 minutes, being careful not to overcook it.

7. Remove the "chips" from the oven and let them rest for a few minutes.

GLUTEN-FREE SUBSTITUTION: Naturally gluten-free!

GROCERY GUIDE: You can find nutritional yeast flakes in most health-food stores. This cheese substitute packs a ton of flavor. Sprinkle it on air-popped popcorn or raw veggies such as broccoli for a tasty treat.

Nutrition information: calories: 150, fat: 6 g., carbs: 17 g., protein: 12 g., fiber: 6 g.

Oatmeal Ambrosia

⅓ cup old-fashioned oats
⅓ cup 2 percent plain Greek yogurt
2 tablespoons raisins
1 teaspoon honey
½ teaspoon cinnamon or pumpkin pie spice
1 tablespoon chopped raw pecans
1 chicken breakfast sausage

1. Cook the oats according to the package directions for thicker oatmeal, using water.

2. When the oatmeal is ready, add the yogurt, raisins, honey, cinnamon, and pecans. Stir well.

3. Enjoy it with a side of chicken sausage.

GLUTEN-FREE SUBSTITUTION: Use gluten-free oats or brown rice.

VEGETARIAN SUBSTITUTION: Follow the recipe for the Oatmeal Ambrosia in the 1,600-Calorie Meal Plan, but omit the sausage.

SHORTCUT: Next time you eat out and they serve a mountain of brown rice, kindly ask for a take-home carton, so you're not tempted to overeat and you have a ready-made supply of brown rice for this easy-to-prepare breakfast.

Nutrition information: calories: 380, fat: 12 g., carbs: 49 g., protein: 19 g., fiber: 5 g.

Wednesday LUNCH

(quick meal) *REVVED* Creamy Chicken Tortilla Soup

Use the second serving of this soup, made for last night's dinner, minus the corn tortilla "chips."

Nutrition information: calories: 390, fat: 13 g., carbs: 34 g., protein: 41 g., fiber: 9 g.

Wednesday DINNER

Turkey Eggplant Parmesan

1 teaspoon unsalted butter

3 tablespoons chopped yellow onion

3 ounces 93 percent lean ground turkey

1 clove garlic, minced

⅓ cup tomato sauce

¼ teaspoon dried basil

⅓ cup 2 percent cottage cheese

⅓ eggplant, sliced into ½-inch rounds (about 2 or 3 rounds)

Cooking spray

Salt and pepper to taste

3 tablespoons shredded Parmesan cheese

2 fresh basil leaves, chopped (optional)

1. Preheat the oven to 350°F.

2. Heat a frying pan over medium heat.

3. Add the butter and onion and sauté the onion for 5 minutes.

4. Add the turkey and continue cooking, stirring frequently, till the meat is browned.

5. Add the garlic and cook until it is fragrant (about 1 minute).

6. Add the tomato sauce and the dried basil and stir the mixture until it is well combined.

7. Remove the turkey mixture from the heat and add the cottage cheese.

8. Place the eggplant slices on a baking sheet. Spray each slice lightly with cooking spray and add a dash of salt and pepper.

9. Top each eggplant slice with some of the turkey mixture, dividing it evenly. Top everything with Parmesan cheese.

10. Bake the eggplant 10 to 15 minutes or until it is tender.

11. Top the dish with fresh basil.

GLUTEN-FREE SUBSTITUTION: Naturally gluten-free!

VEGETARIAN SUBSTITUTION: Replace the ground turkey with vegetarian ground "turkey."

Nutrition information: calories: 380, fat: 14 g., carbs: 27 g., protein: 42 g., fiber: 9 g.

Wednesday SNACK

Tomato and Cucumber Crackers

3 woven whole-wheat crackers (such as Triscuits)
1 tablespoon whipped cream cheese or goat cheese
3 thin tomato slices (about ½ Roma tomato)
3 cucumber rounds
Dash of dill (fresh or dried)

1. Spread the cream cheese evenly over the crackers.

2. Top each cracker with a tomato slice, a cucumber slice, and some dill.

GLUTEN-FREE SUBSTITUTION: Replace the wheat crackers with 5 gluten-free crackers, such as Nut Thins.

Nutrition information: calories: 110, fat: 6 g., carbs: 13 g., protein: 3 g., fiber: 3 g.

Grain-Free Banana-Blueberry Pancakes

1 banana
1 tablespoon almond butter
1 egg
1 egg white
½ tablespoon unsalted butter
⅓ cup frozen blueberries, heated
Dash of cinnamon

1. Heat a frying pan over medium heat.

2. In a bowl, mash the banana with a fork.

3. Add the almond butter and stir the mixture until it is well combined.

4. Add the egg and egg white and incorporate them until the batter is well blended.

5. Melt the butter in the hot pan. Form pancakes using a ¼-cup measure.

6. Flip each pancake after 3 minutes or when bubbles form and cook the other side an additional 3 minutes or until the pancake is golden brown.

7. Top the pancakes with the heated blueberries mixed with cinnamon.

GLUTEN-FREE SUBSTITUTION: Naturally gluten-free!

Nutrition information: calories: 360, fat: 20 g., carbs: 37 g., protein: 15 g., fiber: 5 g.

Egg Salad

4 large eggs
2½ tablespoons 2 percent plain Greek yogurt
¼ cup chopped celery
1 teaspoon Dijon mustard
Dash of paprika
Salt and pepper to taste
2 romaine lettuce leaves
1 pear (optional)

1. Hard-boil the eggs (save 1 for Saturday's breakfast).

2. Peel the 3 remaining eggs; remove the yolk from one and discard it.

3. Place the 2 whole peeled eggs and the 1 egg white in a bowl and mash the eggs with a fork into bite-size pieces.

4. Add to the eggs the yogurt, celery, mustard, paprika, and salt and pepper. Mix well.

5. Serve the egg salad in the romaine leaves and enjoy with a side of fruit, such as a pear.

GLUTEN-FREE SUBSTITUTION: Naturally gluten-free!

Nutrition information: calories: 280, fat: 9 g., carbs: 35 g., protein: 20 g., fiber: 8 g.

Shrimp Tacos with Pineapple Salsa

6 ounces shrimp, peeled and deveined
Salt and pepper to taste
½ tablespoon coconut oil
2 corn tortillas, warmed

SALSA
¾ cup chopped pineapple
¾ cup chopped red bell pepper
3 tablespoons chopped red onion
3 tablespoons freshly chopped cilantro
1½ tablespoons lime juice
1 teaspoon extra-virgin olive oil

1. Place the pineapple, bell pepper, onion, and cilantro in a bowl. Add the lime juice and olive oil and toss the salsa ingredients gently until they are well combined.

2. Heat a frying pan over medium heat.

3. Pat the shrimp dry with a paper towel and add a dash of salt and pepper.

4. Add the coconut oil and the shrimp to the pan and cook the shrimp until they are pink and opaque (about 2 to 3 minutes). Place the shrimp in the warmed corn tortillas.

5. Set aside ½ cup of the pineapple salsa for tomorrow's snack. Use the remaining salsa to top each taco.

GLUTEN-FREE SUBSTITUTION: Naturally gluten-free!

VEGETARIAN SUBSTITUTION: Replace the shrimp with ½ cup canned black beans.

Nutrition information: calories: 400, fat: 14 g., carbs: 42 g., protein: 27 g., fiber: 5 g

Turkey, Apple, and Cheese "Sandwich"

½ apple, sliced vertically into 2¼-inch slices
1 ounce turkey luncheon meat
2 tablespoons shredded Parmesan cheese

1. Top each apple slice with some turkey and Parmesan cheese.

2. Optional: Heat the "sandwich" portions in the microwave for 30 seconds until the cheese melts.

GLUTEN-FREE SUBSTITUTION: Naturally gluten-free!

VEGETARIAN SUBSTITUTION: Omit the turkey and increase the amount of cheese to ¼ cup.

Nutrition information: calories: 130, fat: 5 g., carbs: 10 g., protein: 13 g., fiber: 2 g.

(quick meal) Whipped Cottage Cheese with Fruit and Nuts

1⅓ cups 2 percent cottage cheese or 2 percent plain Greek yogurt
2 tablespoons lemon juice
4 teaspoons maple syrup
¾ cup sliced strawberries
¼ teaspoon cinnamon (optional)
2 tablespoons chopped raw walnuts or pecans

1. Place the cottage cheese in a food processor and pulse until it is smooth.

2. Add the lemon juice and maple syrup and pulse until the mixture is well incorporated.

3. Store ⅓ cup of the cottage cheese mixture in the refrigerator for Saturday's snack.

4. Place the remaining cottage cheese mixture in a serving bowl and top with the strawberries, cinnamon, and chopped nuts.

GLUTEN-FREE SUBSTITUTION: Naturally gluten-free!

FLAVOR TIP: Lemon lover? For extra flavor, stir ½ teaspoon lemon zest into the cottage cheese mixture.

NUTRITION TIP: Walnuts are an excellent source of the healthy omega-3 fat alpha-linolenic acid (ALA). ALA has been shown to help reduce inflammation and the risk of heart disease.

Nutrition information: calories: 380, fat: 15 g., carbs: 34 g., protein: 30 g., fiber: 3 g.

Friday LUNCH

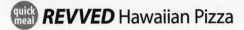 **REVVED** Hawaiian Pizza

3 tablespoons tomato sauce
1 sprouted whole-grain pita
⅓ teaspoon dried basil
5 baby spinach leaves, torn into bite-size pieces
2 ounces turkey luncheon meat or lean ham
¼ cup sliced pineapple chunks
3 tablespoons shredded Parmesan cheese
Dash of oregano
2 fresh basil leaves, chopped (optional)

1. Spread the tomato sauce over the pita.

2. Sprinkle the dried basil over the sauce.

3. Top the sauce with the spinach, sliced turkey, and the sliced pineapple chunks.

4. Sprinkle the pizza with the Parmesan cheese and a dash of oregano.

5. Cook the pizza in a toaster oven or under the broiler until the cheese melts.

6. Top it with the optional fresh basil.

GLUTEN-FREE SUBSTITUTION: Replace the pita with a gluten-free brown-rice tortilla.

VEGETARIAN SUBSTITUTION: Replace the turkey with ¼ cup canned white beans.

NUTRITION TIP: Watching your waistline doesn't mean you have to forgo all of your favorite foods. This tasty pizza has fewer than 300 calories and is a great source of protein and fiber. Compared to a deep-dish takeout, you save over 800 calories by making your pizza at home.

Nutrition information: calories: 290, fat: 9 g., carbs: 29 g., protein: 28 g., fiber: 4 g.

Seared Sea Scallops with Roasted Garlic Potatoes and Green Beans

1 small potato, diced
1 teaspoon extra-virgin olive oil
⅓ teaspoon garlic powder
Salt and pepper to taste
8 ounces sea scallops, rinsed, with small muscle removed
½ tablespoon unsalted butter
1 cup frozen green beans

1. Preheat the oven to 400°F.

2. Toss the potatoes in the olive oil and sprinkle them with the garlic powder, salt, and pepper.

3. Place the potatoes on a baking sheet and roast them for 10 minutes; flip them and roast them for an additional 10 minutes.

4. Heat a frying pan over medium-high heat.

5. Pat the scallops dry with a paper towel. Season them with salt and pepper.

6. Add the butter to the hot pan.

7. Sear the scallops 90 seconds to 2 minutes, depending on their thickness. Flip them and cook them an additional 90 seconds to 2 minutes or until they are translucent. Set them aside.

8. Steam or microwave the beans.

9. Serve the scallops with the potatoes and green beans.

GLUTEN-FREE SUBSTITUTION: Naturally gluten-free!

VEGETARIAN SUBSTITUTION: Replace the scallops with a vegetarian patty, such as a Sunshine Burger.

NUTRITION TIP: Potatoes get a bad rap. Yes, French fries are not the best choice when trying to watch your waistline, but a small baked potato (about the size of racquetball) is an excellent source of potassium (almost twice as much as a small banana). Potatoes are high on the glycemic index, which means they make the perfect side dish for your postworkout meal when paired with an excellent source of protein (such as scallops or any seafood of your choice).

Nutrition information: calories: 420, fat: 12 g., carbs: 44 g., protein: 32 g., fiber: 6 g.

Friday SNACK

quick meal Black Bean and Pineapple Salad

½ cup pineapple salsa (from Thursday's dinner)
¼ cup canned black beans, rinsed

Combine the salsa and black beans and toss them gently.

GLUTEN-FREE SUBSTITUTION: Naturally gluten-free!

Nutrition information: calories: 100, fat: 2 g., carbs: 18 g., protein: 4 g., fiber: 4 g.

Saturday BREAKFAST

(quick meal) On-the-Go Breakfast

1 tablespoon almond butter
½ sprouted whole-grain English muffin or 1 slice sprouted whole-grain bread,
    toasted
1 hard-boiled egg (from Thursday's lunch)
1 small apple
1 8-ounce 2 percent milk latte or milk

1. Spread the almond butter on the toast.
2. Enjoy the toast with the egg, apple, and latte.

GLUTEN-FREE SUBSTITUTION: Replace the bread with a slice of gluten-free bread or a tortilla.

> **NUTRITION TIP:** Avoid sugar-free syrups and flavorings when ordering your favorite coffee beverages. The latest research shows that artificial sweeteners may not help you achieve your ideal body weight. Experts believe that artificial sweeteners may alter our perception of sweetness and actually cause more carbohydrate cravings.[9] If you really need a little flavor in your coffee beverage, wean yourself off sweeteners and try adding spices such as nutmeg, cinnamon, or pumpkin pie spice—or better yet, become a tea drinker!

Nutrition information: calories: 410, fat: 17 g., carbs: 48 g., protein: 20 g., fiber: 8 g.

Portobello Mushroom and Spinach Dip with Pita "Chips"

For optimal flavor, marinate the mushroom for at least 2 hours.

1 portobello mushroom

1 teaspoon pine nuts

1 teaspoon unsalted butter

2 cups baby spinach

1/3 cup 2 percent cottage cheese

1/2 ounce goat cheese

1 1/2 tablespoons chopped sundried tomato packed in olive oil

Salt and pepper to taste

1/2 sprouted whole-grain pita, toasted

MARINADE

1 teaspoon balsamic vinegar

1 teaspoon honey

1 teaspoon Dijon mustard

Dash of cumin

1 tablespoon extra-virgin olive oil

1 tablespoon water

Salt and pepper to taste

1. Clean and stem the mushroom. Remove the gills with a spoon.

2. Mix all the marinade ingredients in a small bowl, then pour the marinade over the mushroom in a glass container, cover, and refrigerate for at least 2 hours.

3. Remove the mushroom and slice it into 1-inch pieces; discard the marinade.

4. In a small saucepan set over medium heat, toast the pine nuts until they are golden brown; set them aside.

5. Add the butter to the pan and sauté the mushroom, stirring frequently; set it aside.

6. Add the spinach to the pan and cook it until it is just wilted.

7. In a medium bowl, mix the pine nuts, mushroom, spinach, cottage cheese, goat cheese, sundried tomatoes, salt, and pepper, stirring until the dip is well combined.

8. Serve the dip with the toasted pita, sliced into 4 wedges.

GLUTEN-FREE SUBSTITUTION: Serve the dip with gluten-free crackers or ½ toasted brown-rice tortilla.

Nutrition information: calories: 320, fat: 18 g., carbs: 28 g., protein: 17 g., fiber: 6 g.

Saturday DINNER

REVVED Turkey Casserole

1 teaspoon coconut oil

½ cup diced sweet potato

3 tablespoons chopped yellow onion

3 ounces 93 percent lean ground turkey

1 clove garlic, minced

¼ cup canned black beans, rinsed

½ cup tomato sauce

1 teaspoon Dijon mustard

½ teaspoon chili powder

¼ teaspoon cumin

⅓ teaspoon paprika

½ teaspoon apple cider vinegar

1 teaspoon maple syrup

1½ cups stemmed and chopped kale

¼ cup water

1 tablespoon raisins

1. Heat a frying pan over medium-high heat.

2. Add the coconut oil and sweet potato and sauté the sweeet potato for 5 minutes, stirring occasionally; set it aside.

3. Add the onion and cook it until it is soft (about 3 minutes); set it aside with the sweet potato.

4. Brown the meat until it is cooked thoroughly.

5. Add the garlic and cook the mixture until it is fragrant.

6. Add the sweet potato, onion, black beans, tomato sauce, mustard, chili powder, cumin, paprika, vinegar, and maple syrup, and stir well.

7. Add the kale, water, and raisins. Cook the mixture an additional 5 minutes or until the kale has wilted, stirring frequently.

GLUTEN-FREE SUBSTITUTION: Naturally gluten-free!

VEGETARIAN SUBSTITUTION: Replace the turkey with ½ cup cooked lentils.

Nutrition information: calories: 390, fat: 8 g., carbs: 55 g., protein: 32 g., fiber: 10 g.

Saturday SNACK

quick meal Whipped Cottage Cheese with Fruit and Nuts

You will have ⅓ cup whipped cottage cheese mixture in the refrigerator from Friday's breakfast.

⅓ cup whipped cottage cheese mixture
½ cup sliced strawberries

Top the cottage cheese with the strawberries and enjoy!

GLUTEN-FREE SUBSTITUTION: Naturally gluten-free!

Nutrition information: calories: 110, fat: 2 g., carbs: 14 g., protein: 9 g., fiber: 2 g.

Sunday BREAKFAST

(quick meal) Protein-Packed Yogurt Parfait with Almonds and Berries

1 cup 2 percent plain Greek yogurt
4 teaspoons almond butter
2 teaspoons honey
½ teaspoon cinnamon or pumpkin pie spice
1 cup sliced strawberries
2 tablespoons slivered almonds

1. In a medium bowl, mix the yogurt, almond butter, honey, and cinnamon.

2. Top the mixture with the strawberries and slivered almonds.

GLUTEN-FREE SUBSTITUTION: Naturally gluten-free!

NUTRITION TIP: Cinnamon, as little as ½ teaspoon per day, has been shown to help regulate blood-glucose levels and promote insulin sensitivity.[10]

Nutrition information: calories: 520, fat: 27 g., carbs: 44 g., protein: 34 g., fiber: 8 g.

Sunday LUNCH

quick meal Tuna Salad with Pita "Chips" and Carrot Sticks

1 sprouted whole-grain pita
5 ounces tuna packed in water, drained
¼ cup hummus
1½ tablespoons lemon juice
1½ tablespoons freshly chopped parsley
1⅓ cups carrot sticks

1. Toast the pita; when it is golden brown, slice it into wedges.

2. Drain the tuna well and place it in a small bowl.

3. Add the hummus, lemon juice, and parsley and mix until the salad is incorporated.

4. Serve the tuna salad with pita "chips" and carrot sticks.

GLUTEN-FREE SUBSTITUTION: Serve with gluten-free crackers or a brown-rice tortilla.

VEGETARIAN SUBSTITUTION: Replace the tuna with 2 hard-boiled eggs plus 2 hard-boiled egg whites.

SHORTCUT: Find a flavorful hummus, such as roasted red pepper, and omit the lemon juice and fresh parsley.

NUTRITION TIP: Tuna is an excellent source of DHA and EPA, two omega-3 fatty acids shown to help reduce inflammation and promote heart health and healthy aging.

Nutrition information: calories: 400, fat: 8 g., carbs: 39 g., protein: 46 g., fiber: 9 g.

Roasted Chicken with Broccoli, Tomato, and Rice Medley

1 cup brown rice
1 rotisserie chicken
2 teaspoons lemon juice
2½ tablespoons freshly chopped parsley
Salt and pepper to taste
7 cherry tomatoes, halved
1⅓ cups frozen broccoli, steamed
4 teaspoons shredded Parmesan cheese

1. Cook the rice according to its package directions.

2. While the rice cooks, remove the skin from the chicken.

3. Cut the breast meat off both sides and set it aside. (The remainder of the rotisserie chicken will be used later for chicken broth.)

4. When the rice is ready, place ½ cup of the cooked rice in a bowl (store the remainder in an airtight container in the refrigerator for Monday's and Tuesday's dinners).

5. Mix the rice with the lemon juice and parsley, and season with salt and pepper.

6. Add the tomatoes and steamed broccoli and toss gently.

7. Top with the cheese, and serve with 4 ounces of the chicken breast.

GLUTEN-FREE SUBSTITUTION: Naturally gluten-free!

VEGETARIAN SUBSTITUTION: Replace the chicken with a vegetarian patty, such as a Sunshine Burger and increase the amount of cheese to 2 tablespoons.

NUTRITION TIP: Chicken is a very lean source of protein that is filling and packed with good nutrition. If at all possible, choose pastured-raised chickens, which have been shown to have higher amounts of vitamins A and E and up to 25 percent more omega-3s compared to chickens fed an all-grain diet.

STORAGE TIP: Place the remaining chicken breast in an airtight container. Do not cut it into cubes or slices; it will be less likely to dry out when intact. If gelatin forms on the outside of the chicken, simply wipe it off. Make sure to use it within three days from the date of purchase.[11]

Nutrition information: calories: 480, fat: 10 g., carbs: 44 g., protein: 58 g., fiber: 8 g.

REVVED Chicken Bone Broth

This is your own homemade chicken broth! Two cups will be used for the *REVVED*-Up Soup for Wednesday's dinner. Store the remainder in the freezer for future use.

Makes about 3½ cups

> 1 rotisserie chicken (remaining from dinner)
> 5 cups water
> 1 tablespoon apple cider vinegar

1. Remove all the skin from the chicken and discard it.

2. Cut the chicken into pieces.

3. Place all the chicken pieces in a slow cooker.

4. Add the water and vinegar.

5. Cook on low for 7 to 8 hours.

6. Strain the broth and store it in an airtight container in the refrigerator.

NUTRITION TIP: Put down that carton of store-bought broth! Take these simple steps and make your own very healthy and healing bone broth. Bone broth is packed with essential vitamins and minerals, such as calcium, magnesium, and zinc! Next time you're feeling under the weather, make your favorite soup with this simple chicken bone broth recipe.

Banana with Almond Butter

½ banana
1½ tablespoons almond butter

Slice the banana into rounds and top each round with a bit of almond butter.

GLUTEN-FREE SUBSTITUTION: Naturally gluten-free!

Nutrition information: calories: 180, fat: 11 g., carbs: 17 g., protein: 6 g., fiber: 4 g.

Nutty Apple Oatmeal and Breakfast Sausage

½ cup old-fashioned oats
¾ cup 2 percent milk
4 teaspoons almond butter
½ small apple, diced
¼ teaspoon cinnamon or pumpkin pie spice (optional)
1 chicken breakfast sausage

1. Cook the oats according to the package directions, using the milk. If you like your oatmeal thinner, add 2 tablespoons water.

2. When the oatmeal is ready, add the almond butter, diced apple (store the remaining ½ apple for today's snack), and cinnamon.

3. Serve the oatmeal with the chicken sausage.

GLUTEN-FREE SUBSTITUTION: Use gluten-free oats.

VEGETARIAN SUBSTITUTION: Add 2 tablespoons almond butter rather than 1 and ½ cup plain Greek yogurt.

NUTRITION TIP: Oatmeal is a natural source of plant sterols. Plant sterols have been shown to help reduce cholesterol levels and promote heart health.[12]

STORAGE TIP: Store the remaining ½ apple (unpeeled and unchopped) flesh-side down on a small plate in the fridge, or if you're on the go, place it in an airtight container with a touch of lemon juice to prevent browning.

Nutrition information: calories: 510, fat: 27 g., carbs: 52 g., protein: 24 g., fiber: 8 g.

quick meal Tarragon Chicken Salad Boats

4 ounces cooked chicken breast (from rotisserie chicken), cubed
⅓ cup halved grapes
⅓ cup thinly sliced celery
¼ cup 2 percent plain Greek yogurt
1½ teaspoons honey
2 teaspoons freshly chopped tarragon
Salt and pepper to taste
3 romaine leaves
1½ tablespoons slivered almonds

1. In a large bowl, combine the cooked chicken, sliced grapes, and celery.

2. In a small bowl, mix the yogurt, honey, and tarragon.

3. Toss the chicken with the dressing until the mixture is well combined, then season with salt and pepper.

4. Assemble the lettuce "boats" and top with the slivered almonds.

GLUTEN-FREE SUBSTITUTION: Naturally gluten-free!

VEGETARIAN SUBSTITUTION: Replace the chicken with ¾ cup canned white beans.

SHORTCUT: Substitute ¾ teaspoon dried tarragon for fresh tarragon. Purchase prewashed and trimmed romaine leaves.

MONEY-SAVING TIP: What to do with extra tarragon? Place it in an airtight container and store it in the freezer for up to six months. Tarragon can be used to infuse oils or for future chicken recipes!

NUTRITION TIP: Romaine leaves make an excellent low-calorie nutrient-dense substitute for bread and crackers. Roll the romaine leaf for a wrap or use it as the base of an open-faced "sandwich."

Nutrition information: calories: 410, fat: 10 g., carbs: 35 g., protein: 44 g., fiber: 5 g.

Thai Turkey Lettuce Wraps

1½ teaspoons unsalted butter

⅓ cup diced red bell pepper

5½ ounces 93 percent lean ground turkey

1 garlic clove, minced

2½ teaspoons soy sauce

2 teaspoons freshly grated ginger or 1 teaspoon ground ginger

¼ teaspoon cinnamon

2 teaspoons maple syrup

⅓ teaspoon crushed red pepper (optional)

⅓ cup shredded carrots

⅓ cup water

½ cup brown rice (from Sunday)

3 romaine lettuce leaves

⅓ cup freshly chopped cilantro

1 tablespoon slivered almonds

1. Heat a frying pan over medium heat.

2. Add the butter and sauté the red bell peppers until they are soft (about 5 minutes); set the peppers aside.

3. In same frying pan, cook the turkey until it is browned, stirring frequently.

4. Add the garlic, soy sauce, ginger, cinnamon, maple syrup, crushed red pepper, and carrots and sauté the mixture over medium-high heat 3 minutes, stirring occasionally.

5. Reduce the heat to medium, add the water, and cook for another 5 minutes until most of the water evaporates.

6. Add the red bell peppers and rice to the pan and cook 1 minute, stirring until everything is well combined.

7. Place the turkey mixture evenly over romaine leaves and top each leaf with the fresh cilantro and slivered almonds.

GLUTEN-FREE SUBSTITUTION: Replace the soy sauce with gluten-free soy or tamari sauce.

VEGETARIAN SUBSTITUTION: Replace the turkey with ½ cup cooked lentils.

GROCERY GUIDE: Invest in high-quality maple syrup. Look for 100 percent Grade B maple syrup; it contains higher amounts of trace minerals and is rich in flavor.

NUTRITION TIP: Ginger is a natural digestive aid. It helps fight nausea and has antimicrobial properties to ward off infection. What to do with leftover gingerroot? Store it in the freezer in an airtight container. Frozen ginger is easier to grate than fresh ginger and can last up to six months. And next time you feel a cold coming on or have an upset stomach, try sipping on a mixture of 1 tablespoon grated ginger, 1 tablespoon honey, and 10 ounces hot water.

Nutrition information: calories: 510, fat: 13 g., carbs: 52 g., protein: 47 g., fiber: 9 g.

Monday SNACK

Veggies with Hummus and Fruit

8 3-inch carrot sticks
8 cherry tomatoes
¼ cup hummus
½ apple (leftover from breakfast)

1. Wash and slice the veggies and fruit.

2. Dip the veggies in the hummus.

GLUTEN-FREE SUBSTITUTION: Naturally gluten-free!

Nutrition information: calories: 210, fat: 6 g., carbs: 36 g., protein: 7 g., fiber: 11 g.

The *Classic* Breakfast

1 chicken breakfast sausage
3 large eggs
1 teaspoon unsalted butter
1 slice sprouted whole-grain bread
1 cup blueberries

1. Heat a frying pan over medium heat.

2. Cook the sausage link according to the package directions; set the link aside.

3. Meanwhile, crack the eggs into a small bowl and, if scrambling them, whisk them with a fork.

4. Add the butter to the frying pan.

5. Once the butter evenly coats the pan, add the eggs.

6. Adjust the temperature to your preferred heat and either scramble the eggs, stirring them with a spatula till a desired doneness is reached, or fry the eggs sunny-side up, over easy, or to your liking.

7. Serve the eggs and sausage with the toast and blueberries.

GLUTEN-FREE SUBSTITUTION: Choose gluten-free bread.

VEGETARIAN SUBSTITUTION: Replace the chicken sausage with vegetarian sausage.

> **NUTRITION TIP:** Did you know butter from pasture-raised cows contains higher amounts of conjugated linoleic acid (CLA)? Diets rich in CLA have been shown to help with weight management.[13]

Nutrition information: calories: 510, fat: 26 g., carbs: 40 g., protein: 31 g., fiber: 7 g.

Shrimp with Jicama and Mango Salad

5 ounces shrimp, peeled and deveined
Salt and pepper to taste
2 teaspoons unsalted butter or coconut oil

SALAD
2 cups cubed jicama
2 cups cubed mango
1⅓ cup diced red bell pepper
⅓ cup chopped red onion
2 tablespoons minced jalapeño (optional)
Juice of 3 limes
1 tablespoon extra-virgin olive oil
⅓ cup freshly chopped cilantro

1. Heat a frying pan over medium heat.

2. Pat the shrimp dry with a paper towel and add a dash of salt and pepper.

3. Add the butter and shrimp to the pan and cook the shrimp until it is pink and opaque (2 to 3 minutes); set the shrimp aside.

4. For the salad, place the jicama, mango, red bell pepper, onion, and jalapeño in a bowl. Stir until the mixture is well combined.

5. Mix the lime juice and olive oil and pour the dressing over the salad.

6. Add the cilantro and toss the salad gently. Reserve half the salad for tomorrow's snack.

7. Serve the remaining salad with the shrimp.

GLUTEN-FREE SUBSTITUTION: Naturally gluten-free!

VEGETARIAN SUBSTITUTION: Replace the shrimp with ⅓ cup canned black beans.

SHORTCUT: Buy peeled and deveined shrimp from the fish counter.

GROCERY GUIDE: Get to know your fishmonger! Fishmongers have a wealth of information on preparing fish and are sure to help with perfect portions.

NUTRITION TIP: Jicama is a hidden gem in the produce section. This tuber is rich in vitamin C and potassium and provides 6 grams of filling fiber per cup with a mere 50 calories!

Nutrition information: calories: 380, fat: 17 g., carbs: 38 g., protein: 22 g., fiber: 10 g.

Tuesday DINNER

Sundried Tomato, Feta, and Spinach Chicken Salad

2½ cups baby spinach
5½ ounces cooked chicken breast (from rotisserie chicken), chopped
½ cup cooked and chilled brown rice (from Sunday)
2½ tablespoons chopped sundried tomatoes packed in oil
4 teaspoons balsamic vinegar
1 ounce feta cheese
2 fresh basil leaves, chopped

1. In a medium bowl, place the spinach, chicken, rice, and sundried tomatoes.

2. Add the vinegar and feta cheese and toss gently.

3. Top the salad with fresh basil.

GLUTEN-FREE SUBSTITUTION: Naturally gluten-free!

VEGETARIAN SUBSTITUTION: Replace the chicken with 1 cup canned white beans.

GROCERY GUIDE: Look for sundried tomatoes stored in extra-virgin olive oil. A little goes a long way; sundried tomatoes are packed with flavor and the additional healthy monounsaturated fat helps you better absorb vitamins A and K from the spinach.

NUTRITION TIP: Balsamic vinegar gives your salads an excellent "tang" while promoting satiety. Research shows that vinegar can act as an appetite suppressant, making it easier to stick to your meal plan!

Nutrition information: calories: 540, fat: 14 g., carbs: 51 g., protein: 54 g., fiber: 6 g.

Dill Dip with Pita "Chips" and Veggies

1 sprouted whole-grain pita
⅓ cup 2 percent plain Greek yogurt
1 teaspoon lemon juice
1 teaspoon freshly chopped dill
⅓ teaspoon garlic powder, or to taste
½ small yellow bell pepper, sliced
½ cucumber, sliced into rounds

1. Toast the pita and slice it into 8 wedges.

2. In a small bowl, mix the Greek yogurt, lemon juice, dill, and garlic powder until the dip is well combined.

3. Enjoy the dip with the yellow bell pepper slices, cucumber, and pita "chips."

GLUTEN-FREE SUBSTITUTION: Swap out pita for gluten-free crackers (about a 100-calorie serving).

Nutrition information: calories: 190, fat: 2.5 g., carbs: 32 g., protein: 12 g., fiber: 5 g.

Smoked Salmon Flatbread

1 sprouted whole-grain tortilla
3 tablespoons whipped cream cheese
1 tomato, sliced
⅓ red onion, thinly sliced (optional)
4 ounces wild smoked salmon
1 teaspoon freshly chopped dill
1 apple, sliced

1. Toast the tortilla in the oven until it is golden brown.

2. Spread the cream cheese evenly over the tortilla.

3. Arrange the tomatoes and onion across the tortilla.

4. Place the smoked salmon on top and finish with fresh dill.

5. Enjoy with the apple slices.

GLUTEN-FREE SUBSTITUTION: Choose a sprouted brown-rice tortilla.

VEGETARIAN SUBSTITUTION: Replace the salmon with ⅓ cup canned garbanzo beans, rinsed. Swap out the cream cheese for 1½ ounces goat cheese.

NUTRITION TIP: Did you know that dill is not only a flavorful herb but also helpful in aiding healthy digestion?

Nutrition information: calories: 450, fat: 19 g., carbs: 46 g., protein: 27 g., fiber: 7 g.

Wednesday LUNCH

quick meal Grab-and-Go Lunch

This lunch will take you back to your childhood. Remember ants on a log? This one doesn't have raisins but does have some extra protein to keep you full!

- **1 tablespoon almond butter**
- **2 stalks celery, cut into 3-inch sticks**
- **4 ounces turkey luncheon meat**
- **⅓ cup grapes**

1. Spread the almond butter evenly over the celery sticks, or use the sticks to dip.
2. Enjoy with sliced turkey and grapes.

GLUTEN-FREE SUBSTITUTION: Naturally gluten-free!

VEGETARIAN SUBSTITUTION: Replace the turkey with ½ cup edamame and 1 string cheese.

QUICK SWAP: On the road? Starbucks sells a Protein Bistro Box that could replace this meal.

NUTRITION TIP: Almond butter has more heart-friendly monounsaturated fats and is higher in omega-3s (alpha-linolenic acid) than peanut butter.

Nutrition information: calories: 400, fat: 20 g., carbs: 28 g., protein: 36 g., fiber: 6 g.

REVVED-Up Soup

Makes 2 3-cup servings

8 ounces 93 percent lean ground turkey

½ tablespoon unsalted butter

1 cup chopped carrot

½ cup chopped celery

¼ cup chopped red onion

2 garlic cloves, minced

1½ cups canned fire-roasted tomatoes

1½ cups cubed frozen butternut squash

1 cup frozen green beans

½ teaspoon dried basil

½ teaspoon dried oregano

1 teaspoon freshly chopped parsley

1 teaspoon whole fennel seed

½ teaspoon salt

½ cup canned white beans, rinsed

2 cups *REVVED* Chicken Bone Broth or chicken stock

2 tablespoons shredded Parmesan cheese (for dinner portion only)

1 slice sprouted whole-grain bread

1. Heat a medium-size saucepan over medium heat.

2. Brown the turkey and set it aside in a separate bowl.

3. Return the pan to the burner and add the butter, followed by the carrots and celery.

4. Sauté the carrots and celery until they are soft (about 5 minutes).

5. Add the onion and cook the mixture an additional 3 minutes, stirring frequently.

6. Incorporate the garlic and cook until it is fragrant.

7. Add the tomatoes, squash, green beans, basil, oregano, parsley, fennel, and salt. Cook the mixture 2 minutes until the spices become fragrant.

8. Add the turkey, white beans, and chicken broth.

9. Bring the soup to a low boil, then reduce the heat and simmer it for 10 minutes.

10. Serve half the soup with the Parmesan cheese and the slice of bread. (Store the remaining soup in an airtight glass container in the refrigerator for tomorrow's lunch.)

GLUTEN-FREE SUBSTITUTION: Naturally gluten-free!

VEGETARIAN SUBSTITUTION: Replace the turkey with ¼ cup lentils (uncooked) and swap out chicken broth for vegetarian broth. Top the soup with ¼ cup cheese. Increase the broth to 20 ounces.

NUTRITION TIP: Fennel seed adds a unique, deep flavor to this soup. It also has been shown to aid in digestion and help reduce bloating.

Nutrition information: calories: 510, fat: 10 g., carbs: 61 g., protein: 47 g., fiber: 16 g.

Wednesday SNACK

Jicama and Mango Salad

Half of the batch of Jicama and Mango Salad made at lunch yesterday is stored in the refrigerator for today's snack.

GLUTEN-FREE SUBSTITUTION: Naturally gluten-free!

Nutrition information: calories: 220, fat: 8 g., carbs: 37 g., protein: 3 g., fiber: 10 g.

Thursday BREAKFAST

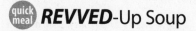 Mediterranean Breakfast Sandwich and Fruit

Even if you are rushing out the door in the morning, you can assemble this sandwich in minutes, and it's a great commuter-friendly breakfast to get you *REVVED* for the day.

> 1 sprouted whole-grain English muffin
>
> 4 ounces turkey luncheon meat
>
> 2 slices tomato
>
> ½ cup baby spinach
>
> 2 leaves fresh basil
>
> 1½ ounces feta cheese or 3 tablespoons whipped cream cheese
>
> 4 olives, sliced
>
> ¾ cup blueberries

1. Assemble the English muffin, turkey, tomato, spinach, basil, cheese, and olives into a sandwich and serve it with the blueberries.

2. If time permits, toast the English muffin.

GLUTEN-FREE SUBSTITUTION: Swap out the English muffin for a gluten-free brown-rice sprouted tortilla.

VEGETARIAN SUBSTITUTION: Replace the turkey with 2 hard-boiled eggs and 1 egg white, crumbled.

Nutrition information: calories: 500, fat: 15 g., carbs: 52 g., protein: 44 g., fiber: 10 g.

Thursday LUNCH

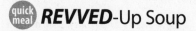 *REVVED*-Up Soup

Half of the batch of *REVVED*-Up Soup made for yesterday's dinner is in the refrigerator for today's lunch.

Nutrition information: calories: 400, fat: 8 g., carbs: 46 g., protein: 40 g., fiber: 13 g.

(quick meal) Parmesan Tilapia with Sundried Tomatoes and Green Beans Almondine

8 ounces tilapia or cod

2½ tablespoons 2 percent plain Greek yogurt

⅓ teaspoon garlic powder

3 tablespoons shredded Parmesan cheese

Salt and pepper to taste

1⅓ cup frozen green beans

Juice of ½ lemon

2 tablespoons slivered almonds

2½ tablespoons chopped sundried tomatoes packed in oil

2 leaves fresh basil, chopped (optional)

1. Turn the oven on to broil; adjust the rack so it is about 6 inches from the broiler.

2. Line a baking sheet with foil.

3. Place the tilapia in the center of the baking sheet.

4. Spread the yogurt evenly over the fish. Top the fish with garlic powder and cheese, and season with salt and pepper.

5. Broil the fish 3 to 5 minutes (depending on the thickness), being careful not to overcook it.

6. Meanwhile, steam the green beans either on the stovetop or in the microwave.

7. Add the lemon juice and almonds to the green beans and toss them gently. Add salt and pepper to taste.

8. Top the fish with the sundried tomatoes and fresh basil.

GLUTEN-FREE SUBSTITUTION: Naturally gluten-free!

VEGETARIAN SUBSTITUTION: Replace the fish with a vegetarian patty, such as a Sunshine Burger.

NUTRITION TIP: Stovetop or microwave? In an *ideal* world, we'd have plenty of time to prepare meals the old-fashioned way. Unfortunately, schedules don't always permit lengthy food preparation. If you are short on time, don't be afraid to resort to the microwave to steam your veggies. Research shows that microwaving may help preserve some of the heat-sensitive nutrients.[14] But if you have the time, grab that steaming basket. Just don't boil green beans in water, because the water-soluble vitamins leach into the water, leaving you with tasteless, nutrient-deficient mush!

Nutrition information: calories: 480, fat: 21 g., carbs: 15 g., protein: 63 g., fiber: 5 g.

Thursday SNACK

Spiced Garbanzo Bites

Makes 2 ½-cup servings

   1 cup canned garbanzo beans, rinsed
   1½ teaspoons unsalted butter, melted, or coconut oil
   1 tablespoon maple syrup
   ¾ teaspoon pumpkin pie spice
   Dash of salt (optional)

1. Preheat the oven to 350°F.

2. Line a baking sheet with parchment paper.

3. Place the rinsed garbanzo beans on paper towels and pat them dry. Transfer the beans to the baking sheet and discard the paper towels.

4. Bake the beans for 35 minutes, stirring them after 20 minutes.

5. In a small bowl, toss the beans with the melted butter, maple syrup, pumpkin pie spice, and dash of salt.

6. Return the beans to the parchment-lined baking sheet and bake them an additional 5 minutes.

7. Let them cool. Enjoy half of them for your snack, and store the remainder for tomorrow's snack. These will keep in an airtight container for up to three days.

GLUTEN-FREE SUBSTITUTION: Naturally gluten-free!

Nutrition information (per serving): calories: 170, fat: 4 g., carbs: 29 g., protein: 6 g., fiber: 6 g.

Friday BREAKFAST

Chorizo Breakfast Burrito and Melon

Makes 2 servings

- 3 ounces chorizo
- 2½ teaspoons unsalted butter
- ⅓ cup chopped red bell peppers
- ⅓ cup chopped red onion
- 3 eggs
- 3 egg whites
- 2 sprouted whole-grain tortillas
- 1½ tablespoons freshly chopped cilantro
- ¾ cup cubed cantaloupe

1. Heat a frying pan over medium heat.
2. Cook the chorizo until it is browned, stirring it occasionally, and set it aside in a small bowl.
3. Add the butter to the pan and sauté the peppers and onions until they are soft.
4. Combine the eggs and egg whites in a bowl, whisk them with a fork, and add them to the pan.
5. Using a spatula, scramble the eggs to a desired doneness.
6. Return the chorizo to the pan and stir the mixture until it is well incorporated.
7. Place half the mixture on each tortilla, add the cilantro, and roll each up into a burrito. Serve one with melon.
8. Once cooled, store the second burrito in an airtight container or plastic wrap in the freezer for Week 3.

GLUTEN-FREE SUBSTITUTION: Choose a sprouted brown-rice tortilla.

VEGETARIAN SUBSTITUTION: Replace the chorizo with 1 additional whole egg and 1 egg white. For extra spice, add ⅓ teaspoon crushed red pepper.

INGREDIENT SUBSTITUTION: Not a chorizo fan? Swap out the chorizo for any flavored sausage.

QUANTITY TIP: One ounce of chorizo is about one-third to one-fourth of a medium sausage link. Although a small amount of meat, it sure does pack a ton of flavor. When making this recipe, consider quadrupling the batch. These burritos freeze well and can be the perfect grab-and-go breakfast when in a hurry. Or share them with the rest of the family—they are sure to be a huge hit!

NUTRITION TIP: Cantaloupe is an excellent source of beta-carotene, an antioxidant shown to promote healthy skin, hair, and aging.

Nutrition information: calories: 500, fat: 27 g., carbs: 39 g., protein: 26 g., fiber: 5 g.

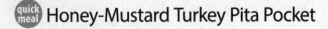 **Honey-Mustard Turkey Pita Pocket**

3 ounces turkey luncheon meat, chopped
⅓ cup shredded carrots
1¼ cup chopped romaine lettuce
5 cherry tomatoes, halved
3 tablespoons 2 percent plain Greek yogurt
¾ tablespoon honey
2½ teaspoons Dijon mustard
1 tablespoon freshly chopped parsley (optional)
Dash of salt and pepper
1 sprouted whole-grain pita
1 orange

1. In a large bowl, combine the turkey, carrots, lettuce, and tomatoes.

2. In a small bowl, mix yogurt, honey, mustard, parsley, salt, and pepper.

3. Toss the turkey mixture with the dressing until everything is well combined.

4. Fill the pita and enjoy it with an orange.

GLUTEN-FREE SUBSTITUTION: Choose a gluten-free pita bread or brown-rice tortilla.

VEGETARIAN SUBSTITUTION: Swap ⅓ cup canned garbanzo beans for the turkey.

GROCERY GUIDE: Pick a pita that is made with 100 percent whole grains. Check the ingredient list. If you see the word "enriched," select a different brand.

NUTRITION TIP: Sprinkle parsley on your favorite salads and soups. Not only will it add delicious flavor and depth but it will also aid in digestion and help with bloating.

Nutrition information: calories: 400, fat: 4 g., carbs: 64 g., protein: 32 g., fiber: 9 g.

Savory Maple-Glazed Salmon with Roasted Rosemary Butternut Squash and Steamed Broccoli

1 cup cubed butternut squash
4 teaspoons butter
1½ teaspoons dried rosemary
5½ ounces wild salmon
1 teaspoon chili powder
Dash of salt and pepper, or to taste
2½ teaspoons maple syrup
1¼ cup frozen broccoli, steamed

1. Preheat the oven to 400°F.

2. Toss the butternut squash with 2 teaspoons of the butter, melted, and the rosemary and place the squash on a baking sheet.

3. Roast the pieces for 10 minutes; flip them with a spatula, and roast them an additional 10 minutes or until they are golden brown.

4. While the butternut squash cooks, heat a frying pan over medium heat.

5. Add the remaining 2 teaspoons of butter to the pan.

6. Season the salmon with the chili powder, salt, and pepper.

7. Cook the salmon skin side down for 2 minutes, flip it up on its side for 30 seconds, repeat the same on the other side, and then finish cooking it skin side down. Add the maple syrup during the last 2 minutes of cooking, using a spoon to catch the syrup and coat the fish evenly.

8. Cook the salmon until its internal temperature reaches 145°F, or to the desired doneness.

9. Serve the fish with the steamed broccoli and butternut squash.

GLUTEN-FREE SUBSTITUTION: Naturally gluten-free!

VEGETARIAN SUBSTITUTION: Replace the salmon with 10 ounces extra-firm tofu.

GROCERY GUIDE: When in season, look for precut butternut squash in your produce section rather than the frozen section for optimal texture. Remember to adjust the cooking time accordingly, depending on the size of the butternut cubes.

> **NUTRITION TIP:** The omega-3 fatty acids DHA and EPA can degrade during the cooking process. To help preserve these healthy fats, make sure to incorporate rosemary in the meal. Research has shown that rosemary helps prevent the oxidation of heat-sensitive omega-3s.[15]

Nutrition information: calories: 530, fat: 26 g., carbs: 40 g., protein: 40 g., fiber: 10 g.

Friday S N A C K

Spiced Garbanzo Bites

Half of the batch of Spiced Garbanzo Bites made for yesterday's snack is stored in an airtight container for today's snack .

Nutrition information: calories: 170, fat: 4 g., carbs: 29 g., protein: 6 g., fiber: 6 g.

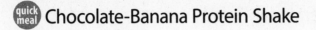 Chocolate-Banana Protein Shake

1 slice sprouted-grain bread
4 teaspoons almond butter
1 scoop whey protein powder
1 cup 2 percent milk
½ banana
1 tablespoon unsweetened cocoa powder
1 cup baby spinach
1 cup ice (optional)

1. Toast the bread and top it with 1 teaspoon of the almond butter.

2. For the smoothie, place the remaining 3 teaspoons of almond butter and the protein powder, milk, banana, cocoa powder, spinach, and optional ice in a blender and blend the mixture until it is smooth.

GLUTEN-FREE SUBSTITUTION: Replace the sprouted-grain bread with ½ banana or 1 slice gluten-free bread.

NUTRITION TIP: Dark cocoa is rich in flavonoids and antioxidants shown to boost heart health, improve insulin sensitivity, and promote healthy aging.

Nutrition information: calories: 490, fat: 19 g., carbs: 53 g., protein: 39 g., fiber: 10 g.

Mediterranean Salad

⅓ cup canned garbanzo beans, rinsed

4 olives, pitted and chopped

1 tomato, chopped

½ cucumber, chopped

2 tablespoons chopped red onion

1 ounce feta cheese, crumbled

1 tablespoon lemon juice

1½ teaspoons extra-virgin olive oil

2 tablespoons freshly chopped parsley

2 fresh basil leaves, torn into small pieces (optional)

Salt and pepper (optional)

⅓ cup seedless grapes, rinsed

1. In a medium bowl, combine the beans, olives, tomato, cucumber, onion, and cheese.

2. Add the lemon juice, olive oil, parsley, basil, and a dash of salt and pepper. Toss the mixture gently.

3. Enjoy the salad with a side of grapes.

GLUTEN-FREE SUBSTITUTION: Naturally gluten-free!

NUTRITION TIP: Although soaking and cooking your own beans is the optimal choice (less salt and fewer gut irritants), canned beans are incredibly convenient. Make sure to rinse canned beans well to reduce their sodium content up to 40 percent.

NUTRITION TIP: A little goes a long way with feta cheese! Just a small amount adds richness and flavor to any dish. This soft cheese has one-third fewer calories and fat compared to hard cheeses such as cheddar.

Nutrition information: calories: 450, fat: 17 g., carbs: 60 g., protein: 16 g., fiber: 10 g.

Cumin-Spiced Flank Steak with Roasted Sweet Potato and Sautéed Veggies

With this recipe, the most labor-intensive one of the bunch, you will do one prep for two meals. For optimal flavor, marinate the steak for a minimum of 2 hours.

1 11-ounce flank steak

MARINADE
⅓ cup extra-virgin olive oil
4 teaspoons balsamic vinegar
Juice of 1½ limes
⅓ cup freshly chopped cilantro
2½ tablespoons honey
1½ teaspoons cumin
Salt and pepper to taste

VEGGIES
1 large sweet potato
2 teaspoons butter
½ yellow onion, sliced
2 red bell peppers, sliced
2 teaspoons balsamic vinegar

1. Place the steak in a shallow glass dish. Mix all the marinade ingredients and pour it over the steak. Cover the dish and place it in the refrigerator for at least 2 hours.

2. Preheat the oven to 400°F.

3. Place the sweet potato on a baking sheet and bake it for 45 minutes or until it is tender.

4. Discard the marinade and pat the steak dry with a paper towel. Let it rest for 10 minutes.

5. Heat a frying pan over medium heat.

6. Add the butter, let it melt, and then add the onion and a dash of salt.

7. Lower the heat to medium-low and cook the onions for 10 minutes, stirring occasionally.

8. Increase the heat to medium, add the sliced peppers, and cook them for 5 to 10 minutes, stirring frequently.

9. Add the balsamic vinegar to the pepper and onion mixture and cook an additional minute, stirring occasionally.

10. Preheat a grill to medium-high.

11. Grill the steak for 4 minutes on each side or until it reaches a desired doneness. (An internal reading of 145°F will produce a medium steak after resting 10 minutes.)

12. Remove the steak from the grill and let it rest at least 10 minutes. Slice the steak against the grain into thin strips.

13. Serve half of the steak strips, half of the pepper and onion mixture, and half of the sweet potato. (Save the remaining steak, pepper and onion mixture, and sweet potato for tomorrow's lunch.)

GLUTEN-FREE SUBSTITUTION: Naturally gluten-free!

VEGETARIAN SUBSTITUTION: Replace the steak with 8 ounces extra-firm tofu. Marinate as instructed. Discard the marinade, and pat the tofu dry with a paper towel. For a crispy texture, make sure to drain the excess liquid from the tofu (placing extra paper towels under the tofu and a heavy kitchen plate on top of the tofu for 10 minutes should do the trick). Sauté the tofu in a separate pan over medium-high heat. Serve with ½ cup canned black beans.

> **NUTRITION TIP:** Why is it important to choose 100 percent grass-fed and finished meats? One hundred percent grass-fed meats have been shown to have higher levels of vitamins A and E and conjugated linoleic acid (CLA), and CLA has been shown to help with weight management. Some meats labeled grass-fed are not 100 percent grass-fed; the cattle are sent to feeding lots for their last month or two. During this time, the CLA content can decrease by 30 to 40 percent.[16] Ask your butcher if your meat is 100 percent grass-fed *and* finished!

Nutrition information: calories: 460, fat: 18 g., carbs: 29 g., protein: 43 g., fiber: 5 g.

Saturday SNACK

Cantaloupe and Greek Yogurt

¾ cup 2 percent plain Greek yogurt
Dash of cinnamon (optional)
1 tablespoon slivered almonds
1 cup cubed cantaloupe

Sprinkle the cinnamon and almonds on the yogurt and enjoy with the melon.

GLUTEN-FREE SUBSTITUTION: Naturally gluten-free!

Nutrition information (per serving): calories: 210, fat: 7 g., carbs: 22 g., protein: 17 g., fiber: 2 g.

Sunday BREAKFAST

Turkey and Sweet Potato Hash

1½ teaspoons coconut oil
¾ cup diced sweet potato
¼ cup chopped yellow onion
4 ounces 93 percent lean ground turkey
½ tablespoon maple syrup
½ teaspoon pumpkin pie spice or cinnamon
½ cup apple, peeled and chopped
Salt and pepper to taste
⅓ cup water
1 egg

1. Heat a skillet over medium heat.

2. Add 1 teaspoon of the coconut oil and the sweet potato, and sauté the sweet potato until it is golden brown; set it aside.

3. Add the remaining ½ teaspoon coconut oil and the onion to the pan and sauté the onion until it is soft; set it aside.

4. Add the turkey to the pan and cook it until it is browned.

5. Return the sweet potato and onions to the pan. Add the maple syrup, pumpkin pie spice, apples (store the remaining apple for Monday's lunch), salt, and pepper, and stir the hash until it is well combined.

6. Add the water and cook the mixture until the water evaporates, stirring frequently (about 5 minutes).

7. Plate the hash, and cook one egg over easy.

8. Serve the egg over the hash.

GLUTEN-FREE SUBSTITUTION: Naturally gluten-free!

VEGETARIAN SUBSTITUTION: Replace the turkey with vegetarian ground "turkey."

STORAGE TIP: Store any remaining apple, unpeeled and unchopped, in the fridge, flesh side down on a small plate, or if you're on the go, place it in an airtight container with a touch of lemon juice to prevent browning.

Nutrition information: calories: 460, fat: 13 g., carbs: 51 g., protein: 37 g., fiber: 4 g.

Sunday LUNCH

quick meal Flank Steak Salad

You will be using the other half of the steak, onion and pepper mixture, and sweet potato you prepared for last night's dinner.

> 2 cups chopped romaine lettuce
> Remaining flank steak (about 4½ ounces cooked)
> Remaining sweet potato, chopped
> Remaining pepper and onion mixture
> 4 cherry tomatoes, halved
> Juice of ½ lime
> 1 teaspoon extra-virgin olive oil
> 2 tablespoons guacamole

1. Place the lettuce in a medium bowl.
2. Add the steak, sweet potato, pepper and onion mixture, and cherry tomatoes.
3. Add the lime juice and olive oil, and toss gently.
4. Top the salad with the guacamole.

GLUTEN-FREE SUBSTITUTION: Naturally gluten-free!

VEGETARIAN SUBSTITUTION: Replace the flank steak with ⅓ cup canned black beans.

GROCERY GUIDE: Flank steak shrinks while cooking, leaving about 80 percent of its original weight. Keep this in mind when grocery shopping and ordering at restaurants.

Nutrition information: calories: 460, Fat: 22 g., carbs: 36 g., protein: 30 g., fiber: 10 g.

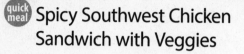 Spicy Southwest Chicken Sandwich with Veggies

2 slices sprouted whole-grain bread or 1 sprouted whole-grain English muffin

1 romaine leaf, torn into 2 or 3 pieces

4½ ounces chicken breast (from rotisserie chicken)

½ large yellow bell pepper, sliced

⅓ cucumber, sliced into rounds

SPICY SAUCE

¾ cup 2 percent plain Greek yogurt

½ small canned chipotle pepper, minced (more if you like it extra spicy)

½ teaspoon adobo sauce

½ teaspoon chili powder

½ teaspoon cumin

1 tablespoon honey

Juice of 1 lime

½ tablespoon apple cider vinegar

2 tablespoons freshly chopped cilantro

1. In a small bowl, mix the ingredients for the Spicy Sauce. (Reserve ⅓ cup for tomorrow's snack.)

2. If necessary, slice the chicken to fit on the bread.

3. Spread 1 to 2 tablespoons of sauce on the bread; top the sauce with the romaine and then the chicken.

4. Enjoy this open-faced sandwich with a side of bell peppers, cucumber rounds, and remaining sauce for dipping.

GLUTEN-FREE SUBSTITUTION: Swap the bread for gluten-free bread or a brown-rice tortilla.

VEGETARIAN SUBSTITUTION: Replace the chicken with a vegetarian patty, such as a Sunshine Burger.

GROCERY GUIDE: Look for chipotle peppers in adobo sauce in the Mexican section of your grocery store. Freeze leftover chipotle peppers and adobo sauce in an ice cube tray and store the cubes in the freezer for up to three months.

Nutrition information: calories: 510, fat: 8 g., carbs: 54 g., protein: 56 g., fiber: 9 g.

Guacamole and Veggies

1 corn tortilla
1 mini container guacamole (100 calories)
8 3-inch carrot sticks
½ cup sliced yellow bell pepper

1. Toast the tortilla and break it into bite-size pieces.
2. Enjoy the dip with the veggies and corn "chips."

GROCERY GUIDE: Check out the produce section for 100-calorie packs of guacamole. These make the perfect heart-healthy snack. Don't worry about waste; these convenient snacks can be stored in the freezer for several months.

GLUTEN-FREE SUBSTITUTION: Naturally gluten-free!

Nutrition information: calories: 190, fat: 9 g., carbs: 23 g., protein: 4 g., fiber: 8 g.

quick meal Triple-B Protein Shake

1 cup 2 percent milk
1 scoop whey protein powder
½ banana
½ cup frozen blueberries
¾ cup frozen broccoli
20 almonds

1. Place the milk, protein powder, banana, blueberries, and broccoli in a blender and blend the mixture until it is smooth.

2. Enjoy the shake with a large handful of almonds (about 20).

GLUTEN-FREE SUBSTITUTION: Naturally gluten-free!

INGREDIENT SUBSTITUTION: Not a fan of broccoli? Feel free to replace it with 1 cup baby spinach. Adding veggies to your smoothie is a surefire way to get your metabolism *REVVED* up for the day.

Nutrition information: calories: 470, fat: 19 g., carbs: 49 g., protein: 37 g., fiber: 9 g.

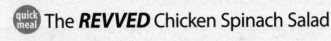 The *REVVED* Chicken Spinach Salad

4 ounces cooked chicken breast (from rotisserie chicken), shredded
2½ cups baby spinach
7 cherry tomatoes, halved
⅓ cup shredded carrots
½ apple, chopped (include any remaining from Sunday's breakfast)
½ cup chopped cucumber
1 tablespoon chopped raw walnuts

DRESSING
½ teaspoon balsamic vinegar
½ teaspoon honey
½ teaspoon Dijon mustard
Dash of cumin
1 tablespoon extra-virgin olive oil
½ tablespoon water

1. Place the chicken, spinach, tomatoes, carrots, apple, cucumber, and walnuts in a medium bowl.

2. In a small bowl, mix well all the dressing ingredients with a fork.

3. Add the dressing to the salad and toss gently.

GLUTEN-FREE SUBSTITUTION: Naturally gluten-free!

VEGETARIAN SUBSTITUTION: Replace the chicken with 2 hard-boiled eggs and 1 hard-boiled egg white, add 1 ounce goat cheese or feta cheese, and increase the amount of chopped walnuts to 1½ tablespoons.

SHORTCUT: *Mise en place* means "putting in place." In the culinary world *mise en place* refers to preparing ingredients in advance and storing them for later use. To assemble meals quickly, set aside one prep day per week to chop vegetables and herbs. Store them in airtight glass containers in the fridge and use them as needed.

GROCERY GUIDE: Look for 100 percent extra-virgin olive oil in a dark glass bottle. Olive oil is subject to oxidation, so exposure to light and heat can destroy this healthy fat.

NUTRITION TIP: Tomatoes are an excellent source of lycopene, a potent antioxidant shown to reduce the risk of certain cancers and promote healthy aging.

Nutrition information: calories: 410, fat: 16 g., carbs: 33 g., protein: 38 g., fiber: 9 g.

Monday DINNER

Maple-Mustard Pork Loin with Roasted Butternut Squash Puree

For optimal flavor, marinate the pork for at least 2 hours.

5½ ounces boneless pork loin
1 tablespoon maple syrup
½ teaspoon soy sauce
1½ teaspoons Dijon mustard
1¼ teaspoons extra-virgin olive oil
1 cup cubed frozen butternut squash
Cooking spray
Salt and pepper
1 tablespoon 2 percent milk
½ teaspoon unsalted butter
8 cherry tomatoes
1⅓ cups frozen broccoli, steamed

1. Marinate the pork in an airtight container in 2 teaspoons of the maple syrup, the soy sauce, the Dijon mustard, and the olive oil in the refrigerator for 2 hours.

2. Preheat the oven to 350°F.

3. Line a baking sheet with foil or parchment paper.

4. Place the squash on the baking sheet, lightly coat the pieces with cooking spray, and season them with salt and pepper.

5. Bake the squash on an upper rack for 10 minutes, rotate them on the baking sheet, and continue cooking them until they are golden brown.

6. Meanwhile, transfer the pork and the marinade to an oven-safe dish. Bake it for 15 minutes or until the meat's internal temperature reaches 145°F. Let it rest 10 minutes.

7. While the pork rests, place the butternut squash in a food processor with the remaining 1 teaspoon maple syrup, the milk, and the butter. Puree the mixture until it is smooth.

8. Place the cherry tomatoes in a baking pan and bake them for 5 to 10 minutes, until they are soft.

9. Serve the pork with the squash, steamed broccoli, and roasted tomatoes.

GLUTEN-FREE SUBSTITUTION: Use gluten-free soy or tamari sauce.

VEGETARIAN SUBSTITUTION: Replace the pork with 10 ounces extra-firm tofu. Cut the tofu into bite-size cubes and cook them on the stovetop until they are golden brown.

INGREDIENT SUBSTITUTION: Not a pork fan? Replace it with skinless chicken or turkey breast.

Nutrition information: calories: 490, fat: 20 g., carbs: 47 g., protein: 37 g., fiber: 8 g.

Plan ahead! Remember to make more *REVVED* Chicken Bone Broth (see recipe on p. 179) for tomorrow's dinner.

Spicy Dipping Sauce and Veggies

You will have ⅓ cup Spicy Sauce in the refrigerator from last night's dinner.

- **½ cup sliced yellow bell pepper (about 5 strips)**
- **5 3-inch carrot sticks**
- **5 cherry tomatoes**
- **4 woven wheat crackers (such as Triscuits)**
- **⅓ cup Spicy Sauce**

Dip the veggies and crackers in the Spicy Sauce and enjoy!

GLUTEN-FREE SUBSTITUTION: Replace the Triscuits with gluten-free crackers, such as Nut Thins, or ½ gluten-free brown-rice tortilla.

INGREDIENT SUBSTITUTION: Feel free to utilize any nonstarchy vegetable with this dip, such as broccoli, celery, cucumber, carrots, zucchini, or cauliflower. Aim for about a 1-cup serving.

Nutrition information: calories: 210, fat: 5 g., carbs: 35 g., protein: 9 g., fiber: 5 g.

The *REVVED* Omelet

This omelet is so packed full of veggies that it is best served "open-faced."

2 teaspoons unsalted butter
3 large eggs
2 egg whites
1 ounce goat cheese
½ cup baby spinach
½ cup diced zucchini
½ tomato, chopped
1 orange

1. Heat a frying pan over medium heat.

2. Whisk the eggs and egg whites in a small bowl.

3. Add the butter to the pan, let it melt, and then add the eggs. Once the eggs begin to firm around the edges, add the cheese, spinach, zucchini, and tomato.

4. Cover the pan with a lid and cook the omelet 3 to 4 minutes or until it reaches a desired doneness.

5. Transfer it to a plate and enjoy it with an orange.

GLUTEN-FREE SUBSTITUTION: Naturally gluten-free!

NUTRITION TIP: Winter fruit options can be limited in certain areas. Avoid dried fruits, as they tend to be easy to overconsume and are more concentrated in sugar, causing a more rapid increase in blood-glucose levels. Check out your grocer's freezer section for a variety of low-glycemic fruits, such as blueberries, raspberries, and cherries.

Nutrition information: calories: 490, fat: 28 g., carbs: 25 g., protein: 33 g., fiber: 6 g.

Tuesday LUNCH

🔵 quick meal Turkey Roll-Up

2 tablespoons whipped cream cheese, goat cheese, or hummus
1 sprouted whole-grain tortilla
½ cup baby spinach
3 ounces turkey luncheon meat
¼ cup chopped tomato
¼ cup shredded carrots
2 fresh basil leaves, chopped (optional)
1 small nectarine, peach, or plum

1. Spread the cream cheese on the tortilla.

2. Add the spinach, turkey, tomato, carrots, and optional basil.

3. Roll up the tortilla and slice it into bite-size pieces or enjoy it as a roll-up.

4. Serve the roll-up with a piece of fruit.

GLUTEN-FREE SUBSTITUTION: Replace the whole-grain tortilla with a gluten-free brown-rice tortilla.

VEGETARIAN SUBSTITUTION: Replace the turkey with ⅓ cup sliced mushrooms and add 1 ounce cheddar cheese.

Nutrition information: calories: 370, fat: 12 g., carbs: 41 g., protein: 29 g., fiber: 7 g.

REVVED Creamy Chicken Tortilla Soup

Makes 2 servings

1 tablespoon unsalted butter

¾ cup peeled and cubed sweet potato

⅓ cup chopped yellow onion

2 cloves garlic, minced

1 cup diced red bell pepper

1 cup sliced and quartered zucchini

1½ cups canned diced tomatoes with green chilis

½ teaspoon cumin

½ teaspoon chili powder

7 ounces cooked chicken (from rotisserie chicken), chopped

2 cups *REVVED* Chicken Bone Broth

½ teaspoon salt

½ corn tortilla (for dinner serving *only*)

½ cup 2 percent plain Greek yogurt

¼ cup freshly chopped cilantro

1 mini container guacamole (100 calories)

1. Heat a medium saucepan over medium heat.

2. Add the butter and sweet potato and cook the sweet potato for 5 minutes, stirring it occasionally.

3. Add the onion and cook, stirring gently, until the onion is soft (about 3 minutes).

4. Add the garlic and stir until it is fragrant.

5. Add the red bell peppers, zucchini, tomatoes, cumin, and chili powder. Stir the mixture until it is well combined.

6. Add the chicken, broth, and salt.

7. Bring the soup to a gentle boil, reduce the heat, and simmer it for at least 10 minutes.

8. While the soup simmers, turn on the broiler.

9. Place the corn tortilla on a baking sheet coated with a touch of cooking spray.

10. Broil the tortilla until it is crispy; set it aside.

11. Remove the soup from the heat, add the yogurt, and stir the soup gently.

12. Cut or break the tortilla into bite-size pieces.

13. Serve half of the soup with all the cilantro, the tortilla pieces, and the guacamole.

14. Reserve the remaining soup for tomorrow's lunch.

GLUTEN-FREE SUBSTITUTION: Naturally gluten-free!

VEGETARIAN SUBSTITUTION: Replace the chicken with 1 cup canned white beans and the chicken broth with vegetable broth.

NUTRITION TIP: Avoid canned soups and prepared soups from your local deli. They tend to be skimpy on the veggies and have an overabundance of cream. Instead, set aside 30 minutes per week to make a delicious and nutritious soup. Aim for at least 1 cup of vegetables per serving and choose a lean source of protein, such as chicken or turkey.

Nutrition information: calories: 500, fat: 17 g., carbs: 47 g., protein: 43 g., fiber: 12 g.

Cheesy Garlic Kale Chips

2 cups stemmed and chopped kale, cut into generous "chip"-size pieces
1 teaspoon extra-virgin olive oil
1½ tablespoons nutritional yeast flakes
¼ teaspoon onion powder
¼ teaspoon garlic powder
Salt and pepper to taste
1 clementine

1. Preheat the oven to 350°F.

2. Pat the kale dry to remove any moisture and place the pieces in a medium bowl.

3. Add the olive oil and toss to evenly coat the kale.

4. Add the nutritional yeast, onion powder, garlic powder, salt and pepper, and toss again.

5. Distribute the kale evenly on a baking sheet, making sure the pieces are not touching each other.

6. Bake the kale 10 minutes, being careful not to overcook it.

7. Remove the "chips" from the oven and let them rest for a few minutes.

8. Enjoy with a clementine.

GLUTEN-FREE SUBSTITUTION: Naturally gluten-free!

GROCERY GUIDE: You can find nutritional yeast flakes in most health-food stores. This cheese substitute packs a ton of flavor. Sprinkle it on air-popped popcorn or raw veggies such as broccoli for a tasty treat.

Nutrition information: calories: 180, fat: 6 g., carbs: 26 g., protein: 12 g., fiber: 7 g.

Wednesday BREAKFAST

Oatmeal Ambrosia

- ½ cup old-fashioned oats
- ½ cup 2 percent plain Greek yogurt
- 2 tablespoons raisins
- 1 teaspoon honey
- ½ teaspoon cinnamon or pumpkin pie spice
- 1½ tablespoons chopped raw pecans
- 1 chicken breakfast sausage

1. Cook the oats according to the package directions for thicker oatmeal, using water.

2. When the oatmeal is ready, add the yogurt, raisins, honey, cinnamon, and pecans. Stir well.

3. Enjoy it with a side of chicken sausage.

GLUTEN-FREE SUBSTITUTION: Use gluten-free oats or brown rice.

VEGETARIAN SUBSTITUTION: Replace chicken sausage with vegetarian sausage.

SHORTCUT: Next time you eat out and they serve a mountain of brown rice, kindly ask for a take-home carton, so you're not tempted to overeat and you have a ready-made supply of brown rice for this easy-to-prepare breakfast.

Nutrition information: calories: 480, fat: 17 g., carbs: 61 g., protein: 24 g., fiber: 7 g.

Wednesday LUNCH

quick meal *REVVED* Creamy Chicken Tortilla Soup

Use the second serving of this soup, made for last night's dinner, with ½ corn tortilla, toasted.

Nutrition information: calories: 420, fat: 13 g., carbs: 40 g., protein: 41 g., fiber: 10 g.

Turkey Eggplant Parmesan

1 teaspoon unsalted butter
¼ cup chopped yellow onion
4½ ounces 93 percent lean ground turkey
1 clove garlic, minced
½ cup tomato sauce
¼ teaspoon dried basil
½ cup 2 percent cottage cheese
½ eggplant, sliced into ½-inch rounds (about 3 rounds)
Cooking spray
Salt and pepper to taste
¼ cup shredded Parmesan cheese
2 fresh basil leaves, chopped (optional)

1. Preheat the oven to 350°F.

2. Heat a frying pan over medium heat.

3. Add the butter and onion and sauté the onion for 5 minutes.

4. Add the turkey and continue cooking, stirring frequently, till the meat is browned.

5. Add the garlic and cook until it is fragrant (about 1 minute).

6. Add the tomato sauce and the dried basil and stir the mixture until it is well combined.

7. Remove the turkey mixture from the heat and add the cottage cheese.

8. Place the eggplant slices on a baking sheet. Spray each slice lightly with cooking spray and add a dash of salt and pepper.

9. Top each eggplant slice with some of the turkey mixture, dividing it evenly. Top everything with Parmesan cheese.

10. Bake the eggplant 10 to 15 minutes or until it is tender.

11. Top the dish with fresh basil.

GLUTEN-FREE SUBSTITUTION: Naturally gluten-free!

VEGETARIAN SUBSTITUTION: Replace the ground turkey with vegetarian ground "turkey."

Nutrition information: calories: 500, fat: 18 g., carbs: 32 g., protein: 62 g., fiber: 10 g.

Tomato and Cucumber Crackers

6 woven whole-wheat crackers (such as Triscuits)
2 tablespoons whipped cream cheese or goat cheese
6 thin tomato slices (about 1 Roma tomato)
6 cucumber rounds
Dash of dill (fresh or dried)

1. Spread the cream cheese evenly over the crackers.

2. Top each cracker with a tomato slice, a cucumber slice, and some dill.

GLUTEN-FREE SUBSTITUTION: Replace the wheat crackers with 12 gluten-free crackers, such as Nut Thins.

Nutrition information: calories: 210, fat: 11 g., carbs: 24 g., protein: 5 g., fiber: 4 g.

Grain-Free Banana-Blueberry Pancakes

1 banana
1 tablespoon almond butter
1 egg
1 egg white
½ tablespoon unsalted butter
Dash of cinnamon
⅓ cup frozen blueberries, heated
½ cup 2 percent plain Greek yogurt
1½ tablespoons chopped raw pecans

1. Heat a frying pan over medium heat.

2. In a bowl, mash the banana with a fork.

3. Add the almond butter and stir the mixture until it is well combined.

4. Add the egg and egg white and incorporate them until the batter is well blended.

5. Melt the butter in the hot pan. Form pancakes using a ¼-cup measure.

6. Flip each pancake after 3 minutes or when bubbles form and cook the other side an additional 3 minutes or until the pancake is golden brown.

7. Top the pancakes with the heated berries mixed with cinnamon. Enjoy them along with a side of yogurt and chopped pecans.

GLUTEN-FREE SUBSTITUTION: Naturally gluten-free!

Nutrition information: calories: 510, fat: 30 g., carbs: 43 g., protein: 25 g., fiber: 7 g.

Egg Salad Pita

4 large eggs
2½ tablespoons 2 percent plain Greek yogurt
¼ cup chopped celery
1 teaspoon Dijon mustard
Dash of paprika
Salt and pepper to taste
2 romaine lettuce leaves, torn into bite-size pieces
1 sprouted whole-grain pita
1 pear (optional)

1. Hard-boil the eggs (save 1 for Saturday's breakfast).

2. Peel the 3 remaining eggs; remove the yolk from one and discard it.

3. Place the 2 whole peeled eggs and the 1 egg white in a bowl and mash the eggs with a fork into bite-size pieces.

4. Add to the eggs the yogurt, celery, mustard, paprika, and salt and pepper. Mix well.

5. Stuff the pita with the egg salad, top it with the lettuce, and enjoy it with a side of fruit, such as a pear.

GLUTEN-FREE SUBSTITUTION: Replace the whole-grain pita with a gluten-free tortilla.

Nutrition information: calories: 390, fat: 10 g., carbs: 56 g., protein: 24 g., fiber: 10 g.

Shrimp Tacos with Pineapple Salsa

7 ounces shrimp, peeled and deveined
Salt and pepper to taste
2 teaspoons coconut oil
2 corn tortillas, warmed
2 tablespoons guacamole or 1 ounce avocado, sliced

SALSA
¾ cup chopped pineapple
¾ cup chopped red bell pepper
3 tablespoons chopped red onion
3 tablespoons freshly chopped cilantro
1½ tablespoons lime juice
1 teaspoon extra-virgin olive oil

1. Place the pineapple, bell pepper, onion, and cilantro in a bowl. Add the lime juice and olive oil and toss the salsa ingredients gently until they are well combined.

2. Heat a frying pan over medium heat.

3. Pat the shrimp dry with a paper towel and add a dash of salt and pepper.

4. Add the coconut oil and the shrimp to the pan and cook the shrimp until they are pink and opaque (about 2 to 3 minutes). Place the shrimp in the warmed corn tortillas.

5. Set aside ½ cup of the pineapple salsa for tomorrow's snack. Use the remaining salsa and the guacamole (or avocado) to top each taco.

GLUTEN-FREE SUBSTITUTION: Naturally gluten-free!

VEGETARIAN SUBSTITUTION: Replace the shrimp with ⅓ cup canned black beans.

Nutrition information: calories: 490, fat: 21 g., carbs: 44 g., protein: 31 g., fiber: 7 g.

Turkey, Apple, and Cheese "Sandwich"

1 apple, sliced vertically into 2¼-inch slices
2 ounces turkey luncheon meat
3 tablespoons shredded Parmesan cheese

1. Top each apple slice with some turkey and Parmesan cheese.

2. Optional: Heat the "sandwich" portions in the microwave for 30 seconds until the cheese melts.

GLUTEN-FREE SUBSTITUTION: Naturally gluten-free!

VEGETARIAN SUBSTITUTION: Replace the turkey and cheese with 1½ tablespoons almond butter.

Nutrition information: calories: 230, fat: 8 g., carbs: 21 g., protein: 24 g., fiber: 4 g.

Friday BREAKFAST

(quick meal) Whipped Cottage Cheese with Fruit and Nuts

1¾ cups 2 percent cottage cheese or 2 percent plain Greek yogurt
2½ tablespoons lemon juice
1½ tablespoons maple syrup
1 cup sliced strawberries
½ teaspoon cinnamon (optional)
2½ tablespoons chopped raw walnuts or pecans

1. Place the cottage cheese in a food processor and pulse until it is smooth.

2. Add the lemon juice and maple syrup and pulse until the mixture is well incorporated.

3. Set aside ½ cup of the cottage cheese mixture for Saturday's snack.

4. Place the remaining cottage cheese in a serving bowl and top with the strawberries, cinnamon, and chopped walnuts.

GLUTEN-FREE SUBSTITUTION: Naturally gluten-free!

FLAVOR TIP: Lemon lover? For extra flavor, stir ½ teaspoon lemon zest into the cottage cheese mixture.

NUTRITION TIP: Walnuts are an excellent source of the healthy omega-3 fat alpha-linolenic acid. ALA has been shown to help reduce inflammation and the risk of heart disease.

Nutrition information: calories: 480, fat: 19 g., carbs: 42 g., protein: 37 g., fiber: 5 g.

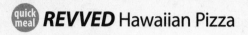 **REVVED** Hawaiian Pizza

¼ cup tomato sauce
1½ sprouted whole-grain pitas
⅓ teaspoon dried basil
8 baby spinach leaves, torn into bite-size pieces
3 ounces turkey luncheon meat or lean ham
⅓ cup sliced pineapple chunks
¼ cup shredded Parmesan cheese
Dash of oregano
2 fresh basil leaves, chopped (optional)

1. Spread the tomato sauce over the pita.

2. Sprinkle the dried basil over the sauce.

3. Top the sauce with the spinach, sliced turkey, and the sliced pineapple chunks.

4. Sprinkle the pizza with the Parmesan cheese and a dash of oregano.

5. Cook the pizza in a toaster oven or under the broiler until the cheese melts.

6. Top it with the optional fresh basil.

GLUTEN-FREE SUBSTITUTION: Replace the pitas with gluten-free brown-rice tortillas.

VEGETARIAN SUBSTITUTION: Replace the turkey with ⅓ cup canned white beans.

NUTRITION TIP: Watching your waistline doesn't mean you have to forgo all of your favorite foods. This tasty pizza has around 400 calories and is a great source of protein and fiber. Compared to a deep-dish takeout, you save over 700 calories by making your pizza at home.

Nutrition information: calories: 410, fat: 12 g., carbs: 42 g., protein: 40 g., fiber: 6 g.

Seared Sea Scallops with Roasted Garlic Potatoes and Green Beans

1 small potato, diced
1 teaspoon extra-virgin olive oil
⅓ teaspoon garlic powder
Salt and pepper to taste
10 ounces sea scallops, rinsed, with small muscle removed
2 teaspoons unsalted butter
1⅓ cups frozen green beans

1. Preheat the oven to 400°F.

2. Toss the potatoes in the olive oil and sprinkle them with the garlic powder, salt, and pepper.

3. Place the potatoes on a baking sheet and roast them for 10 minutes; flip them and roast them for an additional 10 minutes.

4. Heat a frying pan over medium-high heat.

5. Pat the scallops dry with a paper towel. Season them with salt and pepper.

6. Add the butter to the hot pan.

7. Sear the scallops 90 seconds to 2 minutes, depending on their thickness. Flip them and cook them an additional 90 seconds to 2 minutes or until they are translucent. Set them aside.

8. Steam or microwave the beans.

9. Serve the scallops with the potatoes and green beans.

GLUTEN-FREE SUBSTITUTION: Naturally gluten-free!

VEGETARIAN SUBSTITUTION: Replace the scallops with a vegetarian patty, such as a Sunshine Burger and ½ ounce of cheese.

NUTRITION TIP: Potatoes get a bad rap. Yes, French fries are not the best choice when trying to watch your waistline, but a small baked potato (about the size of racquetball) is an excellent source of potassium (almost twice as much as a small banana). Potatoes are high on the glycemic index, which means they make the perfect side dish for your postworkout meal when paired with an excellent source of protein (such as scallops or any seafood of your choice).

Nutrition information: calories: 490, fat: 14 g., carbs: 50 g., protein: 40 g., fiber: 7 g.

Friday SNACK

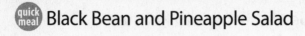 Black Bean and Pineapple Salad

> ½ cup pineapple salsa (from Thursday's dinner)
> ½ cup canned black beans, rinsed
> 1 corn tortilla, toasted

1. Combine the salsa and black beans and toss them gently.

2. Serve the salsa with the tortilla, toasted and cut into "chips."

GLUTEN-FREE SUBSTITUTION: Naturally gluten-free!

Nutrition information: calories: 210, fat: 3 g., carbs: 37 g., protein: 8 g., fiber: 8 g.

Saturday BREAKFAST

On-the-Go Breakfast

> 1½ tablespoons almond butter
> 1 slice sprouted whole-grain bread or ½ sprouted whole-grain English muffin, toasted
> 1 hard-boiled egg (from Thursday's lunch)
> 1 small apple
> 1 12-ounce 2 percent milk latte or milk

1. Spread the almond butter on the toast.

2. Enjoy the toast with the egg, apple, and latte.

GLUTEN-FREE SUBSTITUTION: Replace the bread with a slice of gluten-free bread or a tortilla.

> **NUTRITION TIP:** Avoid sugar-free syrups and flavorings when ordering your favorite coffee beverages. The latest research shows that artificial sweeteners may not help you achieve your ideal body weight. Experts believe that artificial sweeteners may alter our perception of sweetness and actually cause more carbohydrate cravings.[17] If you really need a little flavor in your coffee beverage, wean yourself off sweeteners and try adding spices such as nutmeg, cinnamon, or pumpkin pie spice—or better yet, become a tea drinker!

Nutrition information: calories: 510, fat: 24 g., carbs: 54 g., protein: 25 g., fiber: 9 g.

Portobello Mushroom and Spinach Dip with Pita "Chips"

For optimal flavor, marinate the mushroom for at least 2 hours.

1 portobello mushroom

1 teaspoon pine nuts

1 teaspoon unsalted butter

2½ cups baby spinach

½ cup 2 percent cottage cheese

¾ ounce goat cheese

1½ tablespoons chopped sundried tomato packed in olive oil

Salt and pepper to taste

1 sprouted whole-grain pita

MARINADE

1 teaspoon balsamic vinegar

1 teaspoon honey

1 teaspoon Dijon mustard

Dash of cumin

1 tablespoon extra-virgin olive oil

1 tablespoon water

Salt and pepper to taste

1. Clean and stem the mushroom. Remove the gills with a spoon.

2. Mix all the marinade ingredients in a small bowl, then pour the marinade over the mushroom in a glass container, cover, and refrigerate for at least 2 hours.

3. Remove the mushroom and slice it into 1-inch pieces; discard the marinade.

4. In a small saucepan set over medium heat, toast the pine nuts until they are golden brown; set them aside.

5. Add the butter to the pan and sauté the mushroom, stirring frequently; set it aside.

6. Add the spinach to the pan and cook it until it is just wilted.

7. In a medium bowl, mix the pine nuts, mushroom, spinach, cottage cheese, goat cheese, sundried tomatoes, salt, and pepper, stirring until the dip is well combined.

8. Serve the dip with the toasted pita, sliced into 8 wedges.

GLUTEN-FREE SUBSTITUTION: Serve the dip with gluten-free crackers or a toasted brown-rice tortilla.

Nutrition information: calories: 430, fat: 21 g., carbs: 41 g., protein: 25 g., fiber: 8 g.

Saturday DINNER

REVVED Turkey Casserole

1 teaspoon coconut oil

¾ cup diced sweet potato

¼ cup chopped yellow onion

4 ounces 93 percent lean ground turkey

1 clove garlic, minced

⅓ cup canned black beans, rinsed

⅓ cup tomato sauce

1 teaspoon Dijon mustard

½ teaspoon chili powder

¼ teaspoon cumin

⅓ teaspoon paprika

½ teaspoon apple cider vinegar

1 teaspoon maple syrup

1½ cups stemmed and chopped kale

¼ cup water

1 tablespoon raisins

1. Heat a frying pan over medium-high heat.

2. Add the coconut oil and sweet potato and sauté the sweeet potato for 5 minutes, stirring occasionally; set it aside.

3. Add the onion and cook it until it is soft (about 3 minutes); set it aside with the sweet potato.

4. Brown the meat until it is cooked thoroughly.

5. Add the garlic and cook the mixture until it is fragrant.

6. Add the sweet potato, onion, black beans, tomato sauce, mustard, chili powder, cumin, paprika, vinegar, and maple syrup, and stir well.

7. Add the kale, water, and raisins. Cook the mixture an additional 5 minutes or until the kale has wilted, stirring frequently.

GLUTEN-FREE SUBSTITUTION: Naturally gluten-free!

VEGETARIAN SUBSTITUTION: Replace the turkey with ⅓ cup cooked lentils.

Nutrition information: calories: 480, fat: 8 g., carbs: 68 g., protein: 41 g., fiber: 12 g.

Saturday SNACK

quick meal Whipped Cottage Cheese with Fruit and Nuts

You will have ½ cup whipped cottage cheese mixture in the refrigerator from Friday's breakfast.

½ cup whipped cottage cheese mixture
½ cup sliced strawberries
1 tablespoon chopped raw walnuts

Top the cottage cheese with the strawberries and walnuts and enjoy!

GLUTEN-FREE SUBSTITUTION: Naturally gluten-free!

Nutrition information: calories: 200, fat: 8 g., carbs: 19 g., protein: 16 g., fiber: 2 g.

1,200-Calorie Weeks 1 and 3

SUNDAY

		CALORIES	FAT (GRAMS)	FAT (PERCENT)	CARBS (GRAMS)	CARBS (PERCENT)	PROTEIN (GRAMS)	PROTEIN (PERCENT)	FIBER (GRAMS)
Breakfast	Yogurt Parfait	410	21	46	34	33	27	26	7
Lunch	Tuna Salad	280	5	16	32	46	29	41	6
Dinner	Chicken, Rice	360	7	18	34	38	43	48	7
Snack	Banana	110	5	18	15	55	3	14	3
TOTAL		1,160	38	29.5	115	39.7	102	35.2	23

MONDAY

		CALORIES	FAT (GRAMS)	FAT (PERCENT)	CARBS (GRAMS)	CARBS (PERCENT)	PROTEIN (GRAMS)	PROTEIN (PERCENT)	FIBER (GRAMS)
Breakfast	Oatmeal, Sausage	420	22	47	41	39	20	19	6
Lunch	Chicken Salad	300	8	24	26	35	33	44	4
Dinner	Turkey Wraps	390	10	23	41	42	35	36	8
Snack	Veggies, Hummus		120	3.5	26	21	70	4	13	7
TOTAL		1,230	43.5	32	129	42	92	30	25

TUESDAY

		CALORIES	FAT (GRAMS)	FAT (PERCENT)	CARBS (GRAMS)	CARBS (PERCENT)	PROTEIN (GRAMS)	PROTEIN (PERCENT)	FIBER (GRAMS)
Breakfast	The *Classic*	420	22	47	34	32	25	24	6
Lunch	Shrimp, Salad	280	12	39	29	41	16	23	8
Dinner	Chicken Salad	370	11	27	30	32	39	42	4
Snack	Dill Dip	130	2	14	21	65	9	28	4
TOTAL		1,200	47	35	114	38	89	30	22

WEDNESDAY

		CALORIES	FAT (GRAMS)	FAT (PERCENT)	CARBS (GRAMS)	CARBS (PERCENT)	PROTEIN (GRAMS)	PROTEIN (PERCENT)	FIBER (GRAMS)
Breakfast	Salmon Flatbread	350	14	36	36	41	21	24	6
Lunch	Grab-and-Go	300	15	45	21	28	27	36	5
Dinner	*REVVED*-UP Soup	400	8	18	46	46	40	40	13
Snack	Jicama Salad	160	5	28	29	73	2	5	8
TOTAL		1,210	42	31	132	44	90	30	32

THURSDAY

		CALORIES	FAT (GRAMS)	FAT (PERCENT)	CARBS (GRAMS)	CARBS (PERCENT)	PROTEIN (GRAMS)	PROTEIN (PERCENT)	FIBER (GRAMS)
Breakfast	Mediterranean Sandwich	380	10	24	46	48	27	28	9
Lunch	*REVVED*-Up Soup	370	5	12	46	50	37	40	13
Dinner	Tilapia, Green Beans	340	14	37	11	13	46	54	3
Snack	Garbanzo Bites	110	2.5	20	19	69	4	15	4
TOTAL		1,200	31.5	24	122	41	114	38	29

FRIDAY

		CALORIES	FAT (GRAMS)	FAT (PERCENT)	CARBS (GRAMS)	CARBS (PERCENT)	PROTEIN (GRAMS)	PROTEIN (PERCENT)	FIBER (GRAMS)
Breakfast	Burrito	410	22	48	34	33	20	20	5
Lunch	Turkey Pita	260	3	10	40	62	22	34	5
Dinner	Salmon, Squash	420	19	41	36	34	30	29	9
Snack	Garbanzo Bites	110	2.5	20	19	69	4	15	4
TOTAL		1,200	46.5	35	129	43	76	25	23

SATURDAY

		CALORIES	FAT (GRAMS)	FAT (PERCENT)	CARBS (GRAMS)	CARBS (PERCENT)	PROTEIN (GRAMS)	PROTEIN (PERCENT)	FIBER (GRAMS)
Breakfast	Protein Shake	380	15	36	37	39	34	36	6
Lunch	Mediterranean Salad	350	13	33	48	55	13	15	6
Dinner	Flank Steak, Veggies	390	15	37	28	31	33	31	5
Snack	Cantaloupe, Yogurt	110	2	16	16	58	8	29	1
TOTAL		1,230	45	34	129	43	88	28	18

AVERAGE

CALORIES	FAT (GRAMS)	FAT (PERCENT)	CARBS (GRAMS)	CARBS (PERCENT)	PROTEIN (GRAMS)	PROTEIN (PERCENT)	FIBER (GRAMS)
1,204	42	31.4	124	41.4	93	30.7	25

1,200-Calorie Weeks 2 and 4

SUNDAY		CALORIES	FAT (GRAMS)	FAT (PERCENT)	CARBS (GRAMS)	CARBS (PERCENT)	PROTEIN (GRAMS)	PROTEIN (PERCENT)	FIBER (GRAMS)
Breakfast	Turkey and Sweet Potato Hash	360	9	23	43	48	31	34	4
Lunch	Steak Salad	360	16	40	33	37	23	26	8
Dinner	Chicken Sandwich	360	6	15	40	44	39	43	6
Snack	Guacamole, Veggies	130	8	55	11	34	3	9	6
TOTAL		1,210	39	29.127	42	96	31.7	24	

MONDAY		CALORIES	FAT (GRAMS)	FAT (PERCENT)	CARBS (GRAMS)	CARBS (PERCENT)	PROTEIN (GRAMS)	PROTEIN (PERCENT)	FIBER (GRAMS)
Breakfast	Protein Shake	400	13	29	47	47	34	34	8
Lunch	REVVED Salad	300	10	30	27	36	28	37	7
Dinner	Pork Loin	390	15	35	40	41	28	29	7
Snack	Dip, Veggies	110	1.5	12	19	69	7	25	2
TOTAL		1,200	39.5	30	133	44	97	32	24

TUESDAY		CALORIES	FAT (GRAMS)	FAT (PERCENT)	CARBS (GRAMS)	CARBS (PERCENT)	PROTEIN (GRAMS)	PROTEIN (PERCENT)	FIBER (GRAMS)
Breakfast	REVVED Omelet	360	22	55	16	18	26	29	4
Lunch	Turkey Roll-Up	300	8	24	41	55	21	28	7
Dinner	REVVED Chicken Soup	420	13	28	40	38	41	39	10
Snack	Kale Chips	150	6	36	17	45	12	32	6
TOTAL		1,230	49	36	114	37	100	33	27

WEDNESDAY		CALORIES	FAT (GRAMS)	FAT (PERCENT)	CARBS (GRAMS)	CARBS (PERCENT)	PROTEIN (GRAMS)	PROTEIN (PERCENT)	FIBER (GRAMS)
Breakfast	Oatmeal	380	12	28	49	52	19	20	5
Lunch	REVVED Chicken Soup	390	13	30	34	35	41	42	9
Dinner	Eggplant Parmesan	380	14	33	27	28	42	44	9
Snack	Cucumber Crackers	110	6	49	13	47	3	11	3
TOTAL		1,260	45	32	123	39	105	33	26

THURSDAY

		CALORIES	FAT (GRAMS)	FAT (PERCENT)	CARBS (GRAMS)	CARBS (PERCENT)	PROTEIN (GRAMS)	PROTEIN (PERCENT)	FIBER (GRAMS)
Breakfast	Pancakes	360	20	50	37	41	15	17	5
Lunch	Egg Salad	280	9	29	35	50	20	29	8
Dinner	Shrimp Tacos	400	14	32	42	42	27	27	5
Snack	Turkey, Apple	130	5	35	10	31	13	40	2
TOTAL		1,170	48	37	124	42	75	26	20

FRIDAY

		CALORIES	FAT (GRAMS)	FAT (PERCENT)	CARBS (GRAMS)	CARBS (PERCENT)	PROTEIN (GRAMS)	PROTEIN (PERCENT)	FIBER (GRAMS)
Breakfast	Cottage Cheese	380	15	36	34	36	30	32	3
Lunch	*REVVED* Pizza	290	9	28	29	40	28	39	4
Dinner	Scallops, Veggies	420	12	26	44	42	32	30	6
Snack	Black Bean Salad	100	2	16	18	65	4	15	4
TOTAL		1,190	38	29	125	42	94	31	17

SATURDAY

		CALORIES	FAT (GRAMS)	FAT (PERCENT)	CARBS (GRAMS)	CARBS (PERCENT)	PROTEIN (GRAMS)	PROTEIN (PERCENT)	FIBER (GRAMS)
Breakfast	On-the-Go	410	17	37	48	47	20	20	8
Lunch	Mushroom-Spinach Dip	320	18	51	28	35	17	21	6
Dinner	*REVVED* Casserole	390	8	18	55	56	32	33	10
Snack	Cottage Cheese	110	2	16	14	51	9	33	2
TOTAL		1,230	45	33	145	47	78	25	26

AVERAGE

	CALORIES	FAT (GRAMS)	FAT (PERCENT)	CARBS (GRAMS)	CARBS (PERCENT)	PROTEIN (GRAMS)	PROTEIN (PERCENT)	FIBER (GRAMS)
	1,213	43	32.1	127	41.9	92	30.4	23

1,600-Calorie Weeks 1 and 3

SUNDAY		CALORIES	FAT (GRAMS)	FAT (PERCENT)	CARBS (GRAMS)	CARBS (PERCENT)	PROTEIN (GRAMS)	PROTEIN (PERCENT)	FIBER (GRAMS)
Breakfast	Yogurt Parfait	520	27	47	44	34	34	26	8
Lunch	Tuna Salad	400	8	18	39	39	46	46	9
Dinner	Chicken, Rice	480	10	19	44	37	58	48	8
Snack	Banana	180	11	18	17	38	6	14	4
TOTAL		1,580	56	31.9	144	36.5	144	36.5	29

MONDAY		CALORIES	FAT (GRAMS)	FAT (PERCENT)	CARBS (GRAMS)	CARBS (PERCENT)	PROTEIN (GRAMS)	PROTEIN (PERCENT)	FIBER (GRAMS)
Breakfast	Oatmeal, Sausage	510	27	48	52	41	24	19	8
Lunch	Chicken Salad	410	10	22	35	34	44	43	5
Dinner	Turkey Wraps	510	13	23	52	41	47	37	9
Snack	Veggies, Hummus	210	6	26	36	69	7	13	11
TOTAL		1,640	56	31	175	43	122	30	33

TUESDAY		CALORIES	FAT (GRAMS)	FAT (PERCENT)	CARBS (GRAMS)	CARBS (PERCENT)	PROTEIN (GRAMS)	PROTEIN (PERCENT)	FIBER (GRAMS)
Breakfast	The *Classic*	510	26	46	40	31	31	24	7
Lunch	Shrimp, Salad	380	17	40	38	40	22	23	10
Dinner	Chicken Salad	540	14	23	51	38	54	40	6
Snack	Dill Dip	190	2.5	12	32	67	12	25	5
TOTAL		1,620	59.5	33	161	40	119	29	28

WEDNESDAY		CALORIES	FAT (GRAMS)	FAT (PERCENT)	CARBS (GRAMS)	CARBS (PERCENT)	PROTEIN (GRAMS)	PROTEIN (PERCENT)	FIBER (GRAMS)
Breakfast	Salmon Flatbread	450	19	38	46	41	27	24	7
Lunch	Grab-and-Go	400	20	45	28	28	36	36	6
Dinner	*REVVED*-Up Soup	510	10	18	61	48	47	37	16
Snack	Jicama Salad	220	8	33	37	67	3	5	10
TOTAL		1,580	57	32	172	44	113	29	39

THURSDAY

		CALORIES	FAT (GRAMS)	FAT (PERCENT)	CARBS (GRAMS)	CARBS (PERCENT)	PROTEIN (GRAMS)	PROTEIN (PERCENT)	FIBER (GRAMS)
Breakfast	Mediterranean Sandwich	500	15	27	52	42	44	35	10
Lunch	REVVED-Up Soup	400	8	18	46	46	40	40	13
Dinner	Tilapia, Green Beans	480	21	39	15	13	63	53	5
Snack	Garbanzo Bites	170	4	21	29	68	6	14	6
TOTAL		1,550	48	28	142	37	153	39	34

FRIDAY

		CALORIES	FAT (GRAMS)	FAT (PERCENT)	CARBS (GRAMS)	CARBS (PERCENT)	PROTEIN (GRAMS)	PROTEIN (PERCENT)	FIBER (GRAMS)
Breakfast	Burrito	500	27	49	39	31	26	21	5
Lunch	Turkey Pita	400	4	9	64	64	32	32	9
Dinner	Salmon, Squash	530	26	44	40	30	40	30	10
Snack	Garbanzo Bites	170	4	21	29	68	6	14	6
TOTAL		1,600	61	34	172	43	104	26	30

SATURDAY

		CALORIES	FAT (GRAMS)	FAT (PERCENT)	CARBS (GRAMS)	CARBS (PERCENT)	PROTEIN (GRAMS)	PROTEIN (PERCENT)	FIBER (GRAMS)
Breakfast	Protein Shake	490	19	35	53	43	39	32	10
Lunch	Mediterranean Salad	450	17	34	60	53	16	14	10
Dinner	Flank Steak, Veggies	460	18	36	29	18	43	34	5
Snack	Cantaloupe, Yogurt	210	7	30	22	42	17	32	2
TOTAL		1,610	61	34	164	39	115	28	27

AVERAGE

CALORIES	FAT (GRAMS)	FAT (PERCENT)	CARBS (GRAMS)	CARBS (PERCENT)	PROTEIN (GRAMS)	PROTEIN (PERCENT)	FIBER (GRAMS)
1,597	57	32.1	161	40.1	124	31.0	31

1,600-Calorie Weeks 2 and 4

SUNDAY

		CALORIES	FAT (GRAMS)	FAT (PERCENT)	CARBS (GRAMS)	CARBS (PERCENT)	PROTEIN (GRAMS)	PROTEIN (PERCENT)	FIBER (GRAMS)
Breakfast	Turkey and Sweet Potato Hash	460	13	25	51	44	37	32	4
Lunch	Steak Salad	460	22	43	36	31	30	26	10
Dinner	Chicken Sandwich	510	8	14	54	42	56	44	9
Snack	Guacamole, Veggies	190	9	43	23	48	4	8	8
TOTAL		1,620	52	28.9	164	40.5	127	31.4	31

MONDAY

		CALORIES	FAT (GRAMS)	FAT (PERCENT)	CARBS (GRAMS)	CARBS (PERCENT)	PROTEIN (GRAMS)	PROTEIN (PERCENT)	FIBER (GRAMS)
Breakfast	Protein Shake	470	19	36	49	42	37	31	9
Lunch	*REVVED* Salad	410	16	35	33	32	38	37	9
Dinner	Pork Loin	490	20	37	47	38	37	30	8
Snack	Dip, Veggies	210	5	21	35	67	9	17	5
TOTAL		1,580	60	34	164	42	121	31	31

TUESDAY

		CALORIES	FAT (GRAMS)	FAT (PERCENT)	CARBS (GRAMS)	CARBS (PERCENT)	PROTEIN (GRAMS)	PROTEIN (PERCENT)	FIBER (GRAMS)
Breakfast	*REVVED* Omelet	490	28	51	25	20	33	27	6
Lunch	Turkey Roll-Up	370	12	29	41	44	29	31	7
Dinner	*REVVED* Chicken Soup	500	17	31	47	38	43	34	12
Snack	Kale Chips	180	6	30	26	58	12	27	7
TOTAL		1,540	63	37	139	36	117	30	32

WEDNESDAY

		CALORIES	FAT (GRAMS)	FAT (PERCENT)	CARBS (GRAMS)	CARBS (PERCENT)	PROTEIN (GRAMS)	PROTEIN (PERCENT)	FIBER (GRAMS)
Breakfast	Oatmeal	480	17	32	61	51	24	20	7
Lunch	*REVVED* Chicken Soup	420	13	28	40	38	41	39	10
Dinner	Eggplant Parmesan	500	18	32	32	26	62	50	10
Snack	Cucumber Crackers	210	11	47	24	46	5	10	4
TOTAL		1,610	59	33	157	39	132	33	31

THURSDAY

		CALORIES	FAT (GRAMS)	FAT (PERCENT)	CARBS (GRAMS)	CARBS (PERCENT)	PROTEIN (GRAMS)	PROTEIN (PERCENT)	FIBER (GRAMS)
Breakfast	Pancakes	510	30	53	43	34	25	20	7
Lunch	Egg Salad	390	10	23	56	57	24	25	10
Dinner	Shrimp Tacos	490	21	39	44	36	31	25	7
Snack	Turkey, Apple	230	8	31	21	37	24	42	4
TOTAL		1,620	69	38	164	40	104	26	28

FRIDAY

		CALORIES	FAT (GRAMS)	FAT (PERCENT)	CARBS (GRAMS)	CARBS (PERCENT)	PROTEIN (GRAMS)	PROTEIN (PERCENT)	FIBER (GRAMS)
Breakfast	Cottage Cheese	480	19	36	42	35	37	31	5
Lunch	*REVVED* Pizza	410	12	26	42	41	40	39	6
Dinner	Scallops, Veggies	490	14	26	50	41	40	33	7
Snack	Black Bean Salad	210	3	13	37	70	8	15	8
TOTAL		1,590	48	27	171	43	125	31	26

SATURDAY

		CALORIES	FAT (GRAMS)	FAT (PERCENT)	CARBS (GRAMS)	CARBS (PERCENT)	PROTEIN (GRAMS)	PROTEIN (PERCENT)	FIBER (GRAMS)
Breakfast	On-the-Go	510	24	42	54	42	25	20	9
Lunch	Mushroom-Spinach Dip	430	21	44	41	38	25	23	8
Dinner	*REVVED* Casserole	480	8	15	68	57	41	34	12
Snack	Cottage Cheese	200	8	36	19	38	16	32	2
TOTAL		1,620	61	34	182	45	107	26	31

AVERAGE

CALORIES	FAT (GRAMS)	FAT (PERCENT)	CARBS (GRAMS)	CARBS (PERCENT)	PROTEIN (GRAMS)	PROTEIN (PERCENT)	FIBER (GRAMS)
1,597	59	33.2	163	40.8	119	29.8	30

The **REVVED** Exercise Rules

REVVED Fiction   "Classic cardiovascular exercise is optimal for fat loss."

REVVED Fact   Performing strength training will result in 40 percent more fat loss.

Here's the research that supports the fiction and the fact. Jeff Volek, an exercise and nutrition scientist at the University of Connecticut, conducted a research study in which he placed overweight people on the exact same calorie-reduced diet. He then broke them into three groups: Group 1 did not perform any exercise; group 2 performed cardiovascular exercise; and group 3 performed cardiovascular exercise plus strength training.

After twelve weeks, the average person in the study lost 21 pounds. People in group 1 lost 21 pounds each. That's good. But 5 pounds were muscle, and only 16 pounds were fat. That's not so good.

People in group 2 lost 21 pounds each, but again 5 pounds were muscle. Kind of blows classic cardio out of the water, doesn't it? "Don't do it" is what I have been saying for almost a decade. The cardiovascular exercisers didn't do any better than the "exercise-free" group.

You will learn later on in this chapter that performing lots of classic cardio may be even worse than totally abstaining from exercise when it comes to weight loss (I'm talking *weight loss* here, not the other health benefits of cardio, such as reducing your risk of heart disease, cancer, diabetes, etc.). Take a look at what happened to Juliette (the wonderful nutritionist who formulated our *REVVED* Eating Plan) with regard to her BMR later in this chapter. Shocking!

But what about the people in group 3? People in group 3 lost 21 pounds, but *none* of the pounds were muscle. Therefore, they lost 6 *more* pounds of fat, not muscle, than groups 1 and 2. If you work the numbers, that's almost 40 percent more fat.[1]

Can you now see why I am so anti classic, steady-state cardio or ever dieting without strength training?

The *REVVED* Exercise Plan

The *REVVED* Exercise Plan is a blend of cardio (in intervals, never steady state) and strength training. This is exactly what research has proven to be the winning formula for fat loss. On the *REVVED* plan, you will never, ever get on a traditional piece of cardio equipment, such as a treadmill, bike, elliptical trainer (remember my opinion on those fabricated numbers), or stair stepper. Instead, you will use interval-based strength training to achieve both the cardio *and* the muscle-building and fat-burning benefits. It's so very effective and time efficient.

Not only did group 3 lose more *fat* but they also clearly enhanced their *REVVED* metabolism in comparison to the other two groups, because they didn't lose muscle. Remember that muscle is the engine of your metabolism, and losing it is the worst possible thing if your goal is permanent weight *and* fat loss.

On the *REVVED* Exercise Plan, you will be using a new product called the *REV*olution Glide, or *REVVED*glide for short. Two individual slides can be used individually for every area of the body—upper body, lower body, and core. They also activate a lot of muscles at the same time, which the fitness industry has termed "compound movements."

By activating many muscles at the same time, you make the movement more intense, which is a critically important yet often overlooked component of this kind of exercise.

The three variables to exercise are

1. **Frequency**
2. **Duration**
3. **Intensity**

What do you do for exercise on a weekly basis, if in fact you do anything at all? I bet you will say something like "I run three times a week for four miles" or "I take yoga class three times a week and spinning class twice a week." Everyone focuses on the frequency and duration of the exercise they do but leaves out the *REVVED* secret: intensity.

Intensity is the key to effective exercise. This is why I previously said that recommendations like "Walk 10,000 steps" drive me crazy, because they are not about weight loss. Instead, they are about reducing the risk of diabetes, heart disease, or cancer, which clearly is a positive. But there is a big difference between "disease prevention" and "weight loss"—don't blur it. It should also be noted that disease-prevention recommendations are predicated on the fact that the people they are meant for are completely sedentary. Sure, something is better than nothing, especially when you are spending all day at a desk or on a sofa, but realize that a little walking has nothing to do with losing weight. Look at it this way. Walk a little and disease prevention wins, but weight loss loses. You decide which game you are here to play and which strategy will result in your definition of success.

The Dangers of Cardio

How many times have I said that the human body is very smart? Sure, when you first start taking walks, you burn a few, and I do mean a *few,* calories. But very quickly your body gets in better shape as it becomes more efficient. With that comes frustration and the belief that the only way to continue to burn more calories is to walk longer, more often, or faster. After a period of time, some become more frustrated when weight loss totally stalls (if they were able to lose any at all) and start to run in a dire attempt to lose weight, since the walking isn't working. In no time, some are running ten, twenty, or thirty miles a week or even preparing for a marathon, all clinging to the belief that the running will work, when it really will not.

Let me be very clear: marathons should be abolished. People *die* running marathons; the statistic is that one out of every forty-five thousand people who lace up and attempt a marathon will die. The first marathon runner, Phidippides, ran twenty-six miles in three hours to Athens to proclaim that the Greeks were victorious. After delivering the news, he promptly died of exhaustion.

Honestly, now. Running? No weight loss (as the research proved), diminished muscles, a decimated metabolism, *and* a potentially early death? I'll pass.

My third book was titled *The Cardio-Free Diet.* The original title of the book was *Cardio Kills,* and to this day I wish we had stuck with that for a far more accurate description of my strong belief that cardio kills. In that book, I outlined the dangers of excessive cardio:

1. **Damage to the spine and joints.** The repetitive pounding of running is brutal on most bodies. Very few runners are able to continue to run for many years due to excessive injury to the ankles, knees, hips, and lower back. Some who begin running to lose weight have to stop in a matter of weeks or months, because the last thing you should ever do when overweight is run and pound out your joints. Ditto with the bike and the pressure on the knees. Although I like the concept of spin class—because the exercise is performed in intervals—you have to be aware that cranking up the tension and then standing up in the pedals is horrible on your body. People clamor for space in spin classes. Skip it. Skip the injury. Doing nothing is actually better for your joints in the long run. (Yes, once again, disease prevention comes with cardiovascular exercise, but at what expense to your joints?)

   What about the elliptical trainer, once again a "weapon of mass distraction"? There is not an ounce of evidence or research that proves hours upon hours of elliptical-trainer use is safe, because the equipment is too young. However, I've asked orthopedic doctors, and they agree that the elliptical trainer *can* cause hip, shoulder, back, ankle, or knee pain. Who said that the elliptical motion comes without risk? Shoulder pain can occur because you have to fit perfectly in the machine to use the arms. The majority of us don't. The knee pain comes from a motion that our knees aren't accustomed to doing. More data is required.

   On a final note, I meet people all the time who admit to having had knee or hip replacement just so they can continue to perform *more* cardio. Does that belief system and subsequent behavior sound as crazy to you as it does to me?

2. **Compromised posture.** Quick, go to the window and watch a runner pass by. Remember your friend Jane with the wrinkled skin who runs all the time? Look at her posture. Is that the kind of round-shouldered, hunched-over, neck-jutting posture you admire? How about the cyclists who spend hours at a time in that damaging, crumpled position? They look horrible when they even attempt to stand up straight, which they can't. You will learn later on in this chapter that you should always perform two strength-training exercises for the back of the body for every one that you do for the front. "Why?" you might ask. The answer is enhanced posture. Work

the back of the body, as it gets neglected. Plus, we are constantly in a rounded posture as a result of living at the computer, driving, carrying kids, grocery bags, your purse, briefcase—you name it. Why use your precious exercise time to make your posture even worse? Use that time to correct it, which you will do with the *REVVED* plan.

3. **Impaired immunity.** After 20 to 30 minutes of cardiovascular exercise, your immunity is enhanced because the exercise

   a. Flushes bacteria out of your lungs, so you are less susceptible to airborne illnesses. It is also believed that cancer-causing cells are flushed out through other parts of the excretory system, such as by sweating.

   b. Speeds up white-blood-cell circulation, so an illness is detected earlier. White blood cells are the body's defensive cells. They can also act as a warning device to signal to immune cells that a virus or bacteria may be present.

   c. Raises body temperature, similar to a fever, which slows or stops bacterial growth and helps fight infection.

   d. Slows down the release of stress hormones.

This is all good. Let's be honest; it's very good (and it will be done as part of your *REVVED* Exercise Plan). But the moment you exercise for more than 1 hour, immunity starts to *plummet*.

Two separate research studies support this theory. In the first study, mice were separated into two groups, one that was sedentary and one that performed 120 minutes of cardiovascular activity (running on a wheel). Both groups were then inoculated with the standard dosage of influenza. After repeating this for three days, more of the mice in the second group came down with the flu than those in the first group, and the mice in the second group also had more severe symptoms.[2]

In the second study, scientists at the University of Illinois broke mice into three groups after infecting them with the flu: The first group rested; the second group ran for a leisurely 20 to 30 minutes; and the third group ran for a punishing 2½ hours The researchers repeated this for three consecutive days until the mice showed symptoms of the flu. It should be noted that this particular strain of the flu is deadly to many mice, and as a result 50 percent of the mice in the first group died. So did 70 percent of the mice in the third group! Of the second group, only 12 percent died, proving that short-duration, moderate-intensity cardiovascular exercise enhances immunity. This truly says a lot about what training for a marathon or any similar punishing, unnecessary, pain-inducing exercise does to your immunity.[3]

No wonder so many marathon runners are sick after the event. This happens because the number of white blood cells, which defend the body from disease, plummets, and the stress hormone cortisol shoots up. I already told you in chapter 2 that stress smacks muscle down—hard. Why perform an activity that you know for a fact results in that much damage?

4. **Dirty lungs.** As I just said, exercise can help flush out airborne bacteria, such as those that cause a cold or flu, but that's not the case if you are exercising outside in polluted air. As I write this book, I'm looking out my window at Lake Shore Drive in Chicago. I see lots of runners and cyclists poisoning themselves as they run or cycle along the lake, which is lovely, next to a heavily trafficked eight-lane drive, which is not so lovely. Plus, the busiest time for traffic is exactly when most are out there, as they run or cycle before or after work when each lane is packed. It's pure poison. You might as well put your mouth over an exhaust pipe and practice the deep breathing I introduced you to in chapter 2.

According to an article entitled "Dying Breaths" in *Men's Health*, when you are exercising outside in a heavily trafficked or polluted area, you are

> *Gulping down alarming quantities of pollution: ozone, carbon monoxide, microscopic particulate matter, sulfur dioxide, nitrogen dioxide, lead, and a witch's brew of other pollutants. By conducting part of your workout at midday along a congested street, you are reducing your lung function, constricting your air passages, courting chest pain, increasing your chances of developing asthma, unleashing free radicals to catalyze carcinogens in your bloodstream, and activating cellular processes that might lead to a heart attack.*[4]

I hope this keeps you from ever performing such a damaging activity, especially when you believe that you are doing something *positive* for your body. When I see people running in Central Park in Manhattan, in the filth of all filth when it comes to air quality, I want to tackle them, shake them, and say, "Please, please stop doing this to your body."

5. **Reduced *REVVED* body.** Cardiovascular exercise does NOT build muscle. Many of you performing cardio are thinking, "This is going to help me build muscle and therefore increase my metabolism," when in truth, it's not. Strength training powers a *REVVED* body. Cardio does not. As I told you, excessive cardio actually annihilates your *REVVED* aspirations.

Juliette Britton, who masterfully created our eating plan according to *REVVED* specifications, shot this to me when I sent her the book for edits:

> Just as a side note, when I was training for a high-altitude trail run (thirteen miles), I had the BMR (basal metabolic rate) breath test, and it was 980 calories! It should have been at least 25 to 30 percent higher than that. And I was a fit twenty-six-year-old at the time. The more cardio we do, the more our BMR is lowered.

6. **A ruined weight-loss plan.** You go out, knock off a couple of calories, and then come home and think (and this is the research, not me)

> "I worked out, so I don't have to move around that much for the rest of the day. I'll just wait for the elevator rather than taking the stairs."

> "I worked out, so I can have some fries with my burger."

Those are two ill-advised behaviors after your supposed activity, but they are natural responses after "doing all that exercise."

But there is a far more damaging response. You see, there is one thing for certain that cardio doesn't kill: your appetite! It causes you to eat more. You are hungrier. Your smart body decides, "If I am going to be made to do that run—again—then I'm going to prep for it." And it increases your appetite, big-time! The theme prevails. You tell your body, "I'm going to make you do that punishing run or aerobics class again," and it says, "Bring it on, baby, but I'm going to be one step ahead of you and fuel up, or maybe even fatten up, so I can take the pain."

Again, exercise is a stress. So if you just take a brisk walk, you don't burn many calories, but you don't stress your body out that much. If you do the crazy, long, punishing runs, you jack up the stress response (hello, muscle-shredding cortisol) and sure, you burn a few more calories, but then your body desperately wants the calories back and ups the hunger hormones.

And you decimate your muscle.

And you extinguish your *REVVED* fire.

And you stay at an unhappy weight.

Let's not do classic cardio anymore. Or better yet, let's say we did and don't (that's one of my favorite expressions). Cardio is not healthy, but the

I believe that for the majority of runners, running is an addiction. As with other addictions, the runner needs *more* frequency, *more* duration, and *more* intensity to achieve the same "high" that less running previously provided. It's a bit like cleansing—again! Think about it for a moment. Don't you know people who fall into this category? Is this you?

The growth of extreme cardio events supports my position. A few decades ago, people would run a charity 5K.

Then it grew to a 10K.

Then it grew to a marathon, 26.2 miles.

Then it grew to an Iron Man—a 2.4 mile swim, followed by a 112-mile bike ride, and finishing with a 26.2-mile marathon—*insanity*!

Then it grew to mud runs, where you run, crawl, or even belly-slop your way through mud pits, bog holes, and rivers oozing with thick, cold, gooey muck. It may even include an obstacle course all covered in mud.

Then it grew to boot-camp-style events, where you crawl, frequently again in mud and other slop, with barbed wire just above your head, so you have to maneuver and hover a few inches over the ground like Spiderman, so you don't tear your head open on the barbed wire.

Then it grew to the mud crawl under barbed wire that is now electrified, so if you do hit the barbed wire, not only does the wire itself tear your head open but the electric shock makes it hurt that much more.

And I don't think we are done yet.

Do you see how these activities are an orthopedic surgeon's dream? Business must be booming. I already know it is for all health-care practitioners (chiropractors, physical and massage therapists, etc.) when marathon season starts. It's crazy. Why should our already overburdened health-care system pay for injuries from such ludicrous, irresponsible activities? Don't smokers pay a premium when it comes to health insurance? Shouldn't marathoners do the same?

majority, the *vast* majority, of those who are weight-challenged are still clinging to the belief that cardio is the answer to weight loss. It is *not*.

At the end of your interval-based strength training, I am going to put you through five intervals of HIT (high-intensity training), but that's to optimize the hormonal response and activate even more afterburn, technically termed EPOC—excess postexercise oxygen consumption.

Finally, a note on the number of calories you burn while performing cardio versus those burned while performing strength training: Over the years, countless studies have shown that cardio does burn more calories, but the problem with these studies is that the way the participants performed strength training was very static and not very active. Have you ever heard the expression "benchhead?" That applies mostly to men who perform a set of a strength-training exercises, then let minutes go by, chat, flex in the mirror, whatever, until they perform the second set. It's a very slow process, the heart rate is not elevated, and very *few* calories are burned. This isn't the way you are going to perform interval-based strength training in your *REVVED* Exercise Plan.

On the contrary, the beauty of the *REVVED* Exercise Plan is that you get both your cardio and your strength training at the same time. It's time efficient. It's less stressful and increases compliance—you stick to this plan because it actually works. It's easier to say "I don't have a full hour to exercise, so I'm going to skip it" than to say "I really can get a lot of *REVVED* benefits in just 32 minutes, so I'm going to *do* it."

Plus, research supports my premise. Christopher Scott, an exercise physiologist at the University of Southern Maine, proved that strength training burns many more calories than originally thought—as much as 71 percent more. That's a huge difference, and he showed that based on the findings that performing just one circuit of eight exercises, which takes approximately 8 minutes, can result in an expenditure of between 159 and 231 calories. That's a lot of calories in a short amount of time![5]

REVVED-Up EPOC

Remember EPOC (excess postexercise oxygen consumption), or afterburn? That represents how much time it takes for the body to return to its original state after exercise, given the "muscle disruption" that has just occurred. You "disrupted" your muscles by asking them to do more than they were capable of in the past. You did so by hitting as close to "failure," as in momentary muscular failure, as possible.

When it comes to strength training, there are three stages of a successful 10- to 12-repetition set

Stage 1: Working Repetitions. In this phase, you are able to perform the movements with relative ease. Your form is intact, you are moving at the "one, one-thousand, two, one-thousand, three, one-thousand" speed on the positive and negative. Using a bicep curl as an example, the positive part is when you contract (shorten) the muscle and curl the weight in your hand up. The negative part occurs when you lengthen the muscle and return the weight to the starting position. You are also breathing properly, with the "one, one-thousand, two, one-thousand, three, one-thousand" pace on both the positive and negative portions of each repetition. This should represent the first 5 or 6 repetitions of your 10-repetition set.

Stage 2: Fatigue. In this phase, it's clearly getting harder to perform the movements slowly and in good form. You may start to shake, and you might want to cheat a bit by using momentum, employing less than desirable form, speeding up the pace, or enlisting other muscle groups to help you continue the movements. Don't use any of those options, especially the one where you enlist other muscle groups. Remember this word: "specificity." You want to stay very specific to the muscles that you are attempting to overload. This should represent the next 2 or 4 repetitions.

Stage 3: Failure. In this phase, you no longer can perform the movements. Your muscles are done, the set is over, you have hit "failure." That's always your goal when performing this *REVVED* Exercise Plan. Failure actually starts the "magic" of interval-based strength training that I continue to reference. This magic includes two very important responses to failure that immediately occur:

1. You have created microscopic tears in the muscles. Don't think that is bad. On the contrary, that is what strength training to failure is all about. The body then springs into action and begins the process of repairing these tiny tears. That process is what requires so many calories on a daily basis for muscle maintenance as compared to fat maintenance.

2. The smart brain thinks and instructs the muscle: "You know, the next time you are asked to perform that activity, I want you to get better at it, to have more proficiency. So while you

are in there repairing those tiny little tears, do me a favor and simultaneously build a little more lean muscle tissue. With more muscle, you will get stronger at that movement."

Presto, you just maintained *and* increased your lean muscle tissue. You just fueled a much needed *REVVED* metabolism while dieting.

I can guarantee that you will lose only fat when following the Ultimate Diet *REVolution*. You will get stronger when following this progressive interval-based strength-training program. It's simple as

Strength Up = Muscle Up

Muscle Up = Your Body *REVVED* Up

With the scale heading down and your strength heading up, you guarantee that every single pound registered lost on the scale is exclusively fat. All your long, lean, calorie-burning, strength-inducing muscle is staying right where it was meant to be. And it not only *feels* great—it *looks* great!

EPOC is what truly fuels your *REVVED* caloric expenditure. Research proves that EPOC can continue for up to 38 hours—that's a tremendous amount of caloric expenditure from one 32-minute, intense, interval-based strength-training session.[6]

REVVED Exercise Speed

As I just mentioned with regard to speed, all exercises should be done to a three count, which means "one, one-thousand, two, one-thousand, three, one-thousand" for both the positive and negative portions of each exercise. That indicates that each set of 10 should take approximately 1 minute (3 seconds on the positive and 3 seconds on the negative equals 6 seconds per rep, times 10 reps equals exactly 1 minute).

I should note that far too many people go too fast when strength training. Not only does doing so increase your risk of injury, but it makes the movement far less effective, because you are using momentum and most likely bad form instead of staying very focused on the specific muscle or group of muscles that you are working. In the fitness industry, we refer to staying focused as the "time under tension," and effective time under tension is what overloads the muscle and makes it respond. And with that response comes *REVVED* benefits.

I will indicate resting times in between exercises. Frequently, after you perform 10 reps on one side of the body, you will go immediately to the other side with no rest. When you are changing the actual exercise, then you may rest for up to 30 seconds, which will give you time to grab a quick drink of water and get into starting position.

Breathing is also essential to an intense, interval-based strength-training program. You generally inhale on the eccentric, or negative, portion of the exercise and exhale on the concentric movement. Going back to our bicep curl, you inhale as you lower the weight and exhale as you curl it up. Breathing instructions will be included in the description of each movement.

Remember all the calming benefits of breathing for stress relief? You will get them while you are performing this exercise plan. Think about it for a moment: Cardio *increases* stress hormones, and although, yes, there is some increase in cortisol with strength training, you are minimizing that response as you focus on long, deep breaths with each movement.

> Note to beginners: You may have to ease into some of these movements. By all means, reduce the range of motion if an exercise is too intense. For example, in the third exercise, the lunge, the directions say to go down until your back knee is about 1 inch from the floor, but that may be too low to start, so use your best judgment. Six inches from the floor may be a wiser option. Also, hold on to a chair, kitchen counter, or any flat, firm surface for each exercise if you need to to maintain good form and balance. In no time you will not need this stability, but I want you to listen to your body and be very smart when it comes to when and when not to push yourself.

You will notice that the *REVVED* Exercise Plan has a theme. You are constantly moving from an upper-body exercise to a lower-body exercise to one for the core (abdominals and lower back). The basis of this style of training is called peripheral heart action (PHA), first originated by Dr. Arthur Steinhaus. His style simply alternated between upper- and lower-body sets. I added the core for obvious reasons. The concept behind PHA is that since you are alternating working the upper and lower body, you don't build up a lot of lactic acid. You don't get that "burn" that is off-putting to many beginners and most people working out in general. In addition to the reduced degree of burn, you get another great benefit: an increased heart rate.

Your heart rate *has* to increase, because you are confusing the heart. When you start with an upper-body exercise (as you will in this plan), those muscles need oxygen to perform the movement, and you therefore ask the heart to pump blood out to those muscles. That's why your heart rate goes up. You therefore have a nice "pump party" of oxygen-rich blood going on in the upper body.

But then, in 30 seconds, you switch to the lower body. "What?" the heart thinks. "Now I need to totally shift course and pump blood down there." That shift is going to require the heart to work harder. Presto, you just took classic strength training to interval-based strength training.

Then, you shift course and tell your heart to pump blood to the upper muscles again, then switch to down, then change your mind—again—and perform an exercise that works your core. Now the heart has to once again work harder to pump the blood to your abdominals and lower back.

Please remember that intensity is your goal when it comes to strength training. The harder you work, the more you activate *REVVED* benefits.

Plus, this style of exercise has been shown to really blast fat. You therefore get the trifecta:

- a good, heart-pounding workout in intervals

- maintenance of and an increase in your lean muscle tissue

- a fat-eradicating workout

REVVED Exercise Enhances Posture

As I just mentioned in the "cardio kills" section, posture is destroyed when you perform classic cardio. The exact opposite will happened when you perform the *REVVED* Exercise Plan, as you will be performing two sets of exercises for the back of the body for every one for the front.

You see, when you strength-train a muscle group, you sometimes (but not always) shorten the muscle you are challenging. Remember all the terrible-looking muscleheads from times past, when body builders didn't know what they were doing and focused on their chests and biceps? These men ended looking like round-shouldered apes with big caved-in chests and big arms. Their chests caved in because they didn't work the opposing muscle group—namely, the back.

If you do twice as many exercises for the back as your do for the front, then you will develop and somewhat shorten the back muscles more. Quick, throw your shoulders back. How does your posture look? I'm sure better. Therefore, throughout this *REVVED* Exercise Plan we will hit all the muscles on the back of your body, namely, the following:

Latissimus dorsi (lats), the long, broad muscles of the back that help create that sexy V.

Gluteus maximus (glutes). Okay, your butt. Did you know that the gluteus maximus is the largest muscle of the body? If you have bought into my whole *REVVED* concept, then it's easy to understand that the gluteus maximus is the most important muscle in the body to stimulate. That is why I love the *REVVED*glides, as they do just that.

Glutes Up (Increased in Size) = Metabolism *REVVED* Up

Also think

Glutes Up = Looks GOOD!

On both men and women, symmetrical legs are attractive. If you are among those misfortunate enough to have been performing excessive cardio, I bet you have overdeveloped your quadriceps, the front of your legs, and avoided working the hamstrings, the back of your legs. By performing more exercises for the back of the legs, you will immediately begin to see the symmetry you always wanted but didn't know how to attain.

I just finished reading a magazine article entitled "Is Spinning Making You Fat?" Clearly you know my answer—yes! The article reported that many women were feeling that their thighs were getting bigger. I'm not at all surprised. Why? Because, as I said earlier, when you crank up the tension of a bike and then stand up and push every ounce of your body weight on the pedals, you are bound to tighten the quadriceps, or the front thigh muscles. When you tighten and torture them to such as degree, you make them shorter and bulkier. Plus, the article referenced the fact that many, many attendees of spin classes often take back-to-back classes and spin for 2 hours a day. Like running, spinning can become an addiction.

Can you even imagine the amount of circulating cortisol attaching to belly fat when you spin? If you want big, bulky legs and a belly to match, I say, "Go spin!"[7]

A technical term I want to introduce you to is "reciprocal inhibition." To explain, let me use a simple exercise again: the bicep curl with a dumb-bell. When you curl the arm up, the actual bicep—the muscle you are challenging—shortens. Look down as you perform that movement when your fist comes close to your shoulder. What happens to the opposing muscle, the tricep, or the back of the arm? It lengthens. That's the whole idea of reciprocal inhibition.

When you perform two exercises for the back of the body for every one for the front, it will enable you to pull your body back into alignment, which we in the fitness industry refer to as resuming the "structural integrity" of the body. Basically, it means putting you back together as you were meant to be.

One more note on posture: Look at how babies walk when they take their first steps. Sure, the first few steps are a little unstable, but then they have perfect posture. They stand straight up, shoulders back, chin in alignment. That's the way we are meant to walk. It's only with everyday life that we lose that perfect posture. Trust me, you will get it back, and just wait until the compliments start coming your way. Posture is truly powerful.

Oh, I always have to add one more. When you take a moment, stand up with improved posture and tuck in your abdominals. What happens? They flatten out. Nice visual. In no time your body will be like that all the time. That will be your "new normal."

A few times I have mentioned not just interval-based strength training but progressive interval-based strength training. Why? After intensity, progression is the second most overlooked variable in exercise. I gave you the example of a very damaging progression in which runners start with a 5K and progress to an electrified mud crawl. That represents a negative progression, much like the case of a person who starts having a few drinks to escape the problems of life and, fast-forward a few years, becomes an alcoholic. Instead, we are going to apply positive progression.

Positive progression must occur with strength training. When you can perform 10 repetitions of the *REVVED* Exercise Plan with ease, you are no longer stimulating your lean muscle tissue to grow. If you keep training with the same intensity, you will maintain your muscle, but remember that as we age, the body naturally loses muscle. We want to keep that from happening. That's why we have to continually challenge the muscle to grow and get stronger.

Once again, women, when you hear me say "grow," I don't want you to conjure up the freaky-looking women who sometimes appear on the cover of fitness magazines, or "Muscle and Fiction," as we call it at my firm. Those are most likely steroid-ridden women employing drastic, harsh tactics with both diet and exercise, and possibly even testosterone and human-growth-hormone injections, to achieve that appearance. No, my goal for you is long, lean, sexy muscle. Guys, yes, as a result of our increased testosterone, we will get some pump, but excessive muscle, even on men, is creepy.

With regard to our plan, here are the most effective tools for applying progression:

1. **Increasing speed.** Start your *REVVED* exercises with a three count, as I've already explained. The easiest and one of the safest ways to apply progression is simply to increase to a four count, then to a five or even a six count. That "time under tension" truly brings on the failure that makes your muscles spring into action. *Note:* For exercises such as the plank, you may simply hold the posture longer, which is what I do myself and with clients all the time.

2. **Lengthening each movement.** As you are predominantly using the *REVVED*glides, you always have the option of using a longer range of motion. For virtually every movement, reaching to a farther distance intensifies the movement. When you see the exercises in the next chapter, you will understand what I am talking about. For some of the exercises, I will actually provide photographs of the progressions.

3. **Eliminating the rest time.** You will see that I have calculated the time for each exercise and included rest time when applicable. As you become both stronger and more cardiovascularly fit, I urge you to eliminate

Back in 2005, I spent the summer with Hugh Jackman while he was filming Woody Allen's *Scoop* with Scarlett Johansson in London. Hugh has been an on-and-off client of my firm since he did *The Boy from Oz* in New York in 2003. The reason we were together in London was that I had to get him ready to start shooting *X Men III* in Vancouver as soon as the London shoot was finished. We worked out together. Hugh said to me on the first day (in his Aussie accent), "You know, mate, I really like it when my trainer works out with me." So, lucky me, I got to lift *with* Mr. Jackman for a solid eight weeks. The reason I tell you this story is that we never, ever worked out for more than an hour. Mind you, we were quickly switching positions. He would do a set of 10 repetitions of heavy back rows, jump off the machine, and then it was my turn, frequently at the same weight. We never stopped, but sometimes, after just 45 minutes, I could tell he was almost done (I know I was), and I would say, "Okay, two more sets, and we're out of here." He nodded, we did it, and that was it.

or at least minimize the rest period. That will further challenge both your muscles and your heart.

4. **Adding a second set.** If you eliminate the rest periods and move from exercise to exercise, you may elect to add a second set. Don't think you have to add the second set to every exercise. Go ahead and pick your favorites, but do try to stick with the "two exercises for the back of the body for every one for the front" rule. If you go over the 32-minute mark, that's just fine. That's the minimum of time I want you to exercise; the maximum is around 1 hour. If you can exercise for more than an hour, then your intensity is too low.

The **REVVED** Exercise Plan

Here is your 32-minute interval-based strength-training *REVVED* plan.

For each exercise, perform 10 repetitions to the three count I explained in the previous chapter. Frequently, you will be performing unilateral movements, which means you will first perform all 10 reps on the left side, then repeat on the right. I urge you to start with the left, because for many of us that's the weaker side if we are right-handed. If you are left-handed, start on the right. That way, you get the harder side done first. I know psychologically that works better for me and my clients and may for you as well.

If you are performing the exercises on the bare floor, I suggest using a yoga mat, or any mat for that matter, to protect your knees. On carpeting, you may not find the need. That's totally up to you.

1. Cat-Cow Warm-Up

Consider this a warm-up exercise to prepare your upper body and core for more intensity to come. You will be using the *REVVED*glides, but you won't be moving them. I just want you to get acquainted with how they feel under your hands.

1. Start on your knees with the *REVVED*glides under both hands.

2. You abdominals should stay tucked at all times, your back should be flat, and your shoulders should be pinched together like a cow's.

3. Slowly inhale—try to feel as if you are breathing through your back—as you round your back up and stretch it out like a cat.

4. Remember that it's three counts on the way out and three counts on the return to the starting position, or the cow.

5. You should feel this throughout your entire spine, from the top of your neck to your tailbone.

6. Perform 10 repetitions total.

———————

This exercise should take you 1 minute.

Take 30 seconds for rest and preparation.

Total time: 1½ minutes

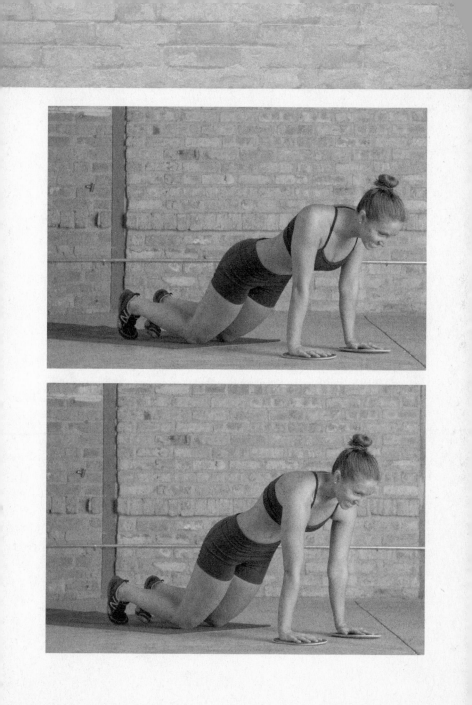

2. Upper Body and Core

You will clearly feel the increased intensity of this exercise in comparison to the first exercise.

1. Stay down on your knees with your elbows on top of each *REVVED*glide, as pictured, and your hands clasped together.

2. Slowly inhale as you remain in the starting position, then exhale as you push your elbows forward on the *REVVED*glides about 1 to 3 inches. Exhale as you return to the starting position.

3. Remember, this is done to a slow count, exactly like the first exercise.

4. You will feel this in your core, shoulders, back, and arms.

5. Perform 10 repetitions total.

Beginner: You may not even be able to move your elbows. Just hold what is a classic Pilates plank (with the exception that you are on your knees) until you feel you are ready for the next challenge. In no time, you will feel your strength increase as you are able to push out farther with each repetition.

Advanced: You may find, in the very near future, that you are able to perform the exercise on your toes instead of your knees, as shown. Just holding it is the true Pilates plank. It's tough but so very effective, and when you are ready to move your elbows, your core will literally fire up and slim down.

This exercise should take you 1 minute.

Take 30 seconds for rest and preparation.

Total time: 3 minutes

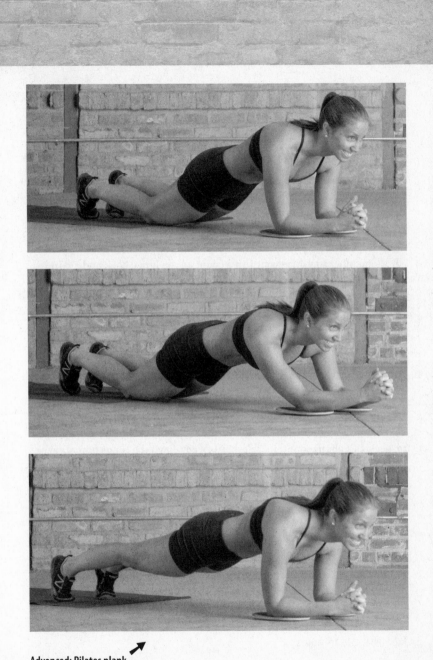

Advanced: Pilates plank

3. Lunges

1. Stand up and place the *REVVED* glides under both of your feet.

2. Stand straight up with your hands on your hips, your feet shoulder-width apart, your toes forward, your knees slightly bent, and your abdominals tucked.

3. Slowly inhale as you slide your right leg back until your knee is about 1 inch from the floor, bent at a 90-degree angle.

4. Hold that position for a moment, then exhale as you return to the starting position.

5. Remember to utilize your three count as you lunge back and again when you return.

6. You should feel this on both sides of your lower body, as the one side is working while the other is providing stability.

7. Do 10 repetitions on the right side and immediately repeat on the left side.

Beginner: You may need to use stability that I alluded to in the previous chapter, so it might be best to do this next to a surface that you can hold on to, such as a chair, counter, or desk. Also, cut down the range of motion so you are about 6 inches from the floor rather than 1.

Advanced: Instead of bending your knee, try to keep the leg straight and go as far back as possible. Hold, then slowly return. You might even go to a four, five, or six count in time, as "time under tension" increases intensity.

This unilateral exercise should take you 1 minute on each side for a total of 2 minutes.

Take 30 seconds for rest and preparation.

Total time: 5½ minutes

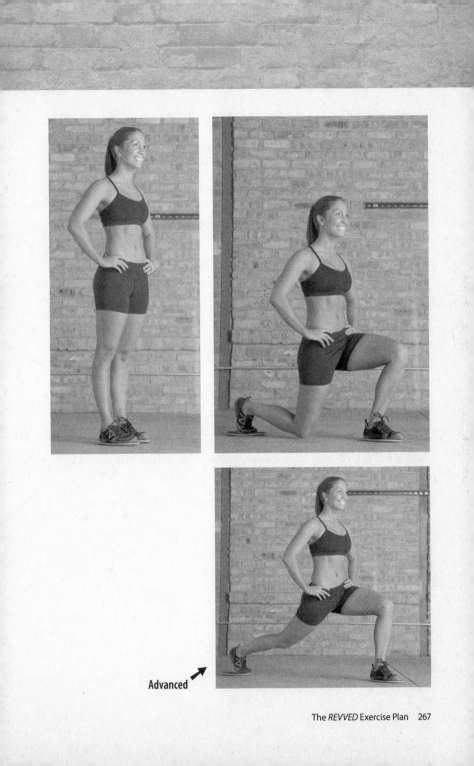

Advanced

4. The Y Back

1. Start on your knees with *REVVED*glides under both hands.

2. Now move the left hand to 11:00, similar to the left half of a capital letter Y.

3. Although this is similar to the first exercise, you are hitting the back and upper-body muscles from an alternate direction. This will stimulate more long, lean, calorie-burning muscles and continue to enhance posture.

4. Inhale as you extend and exhale as you bring your hand back to the starting position.

5. Do 10 repetitions and immediately repeat on the right side, moving the right hand to about 1:00, the right half of the letter Y.

6. Once again, you will feel this in both the upper body and the core as you stabilize your lower body.

Beginner: As with the first movement, you may elect to move only about 6 inches toward the 11:00 position.

Advanced: Try to extend as far out as possible with each repetition and/or increase from a three count to a four, five, or six count.

Superadvanced: Come up onto your toes and start the exercise from a push-up position.

This unilateral exercise should take you 1 minute on each side for a total of 2 minutes.

Take 30 seconds for rest and preparation.

Total time: 8 minutes

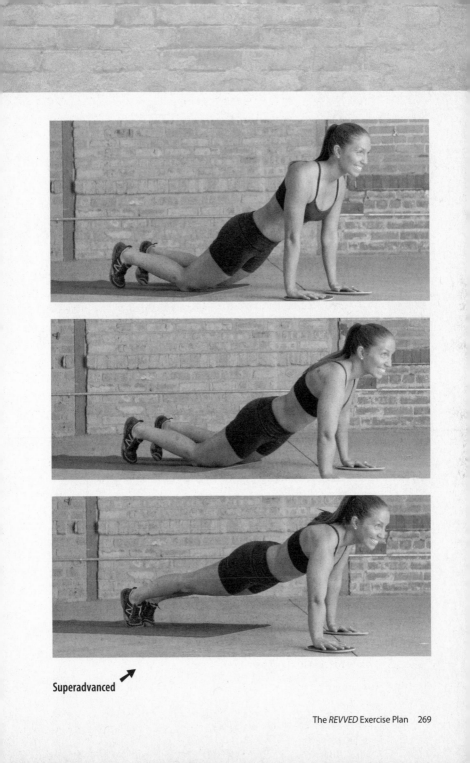

Superadvanced

5. Side Lunges

1. Stand up and place the *REVVED*glides under both your feet.

2. Stand straight up with your hands on your hips, your feet shoulder-width apart, your toes forward, your knees slightly bent, and your abdominals tucked.

3. Slowly inhale as you slide your left leg to the left until it is fully extended.

4. Your right leg will bend to about 90 degrees, but make sure your right knee does not pass your right toe.

5. Hold that position for a moment, then exhale as you return to the starting position.

6. Remember to utilize your three count as you lunge to the side and again when you return.

7. You should feel this on both sides of your lower body, as the one side is working while the other is providing stability.

8. Do 10 repetitions and immediately repeat on the other side.

Beginner: For stability, do this exercise next to a surface that you can hold on to, such as a chair, counter, or desk. Also, cut down the range of motion so you do not extend out as far.

Advanced: Try to go as far to the side as possible. Hold, then slowly return. You might even go to a four, five or six count in time, as "time under tension" increases intensity.

Superadvanced: Extend your arms straight out in front of you. By changing your center of gravity, you make the exercise even more intense.

This unilateral exercise should take you 1 minute on each side for a total of 2 minutes.

Take 30 seconds for rest and preparation.

Total time: 10½ minutes

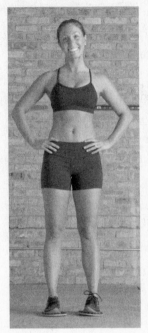

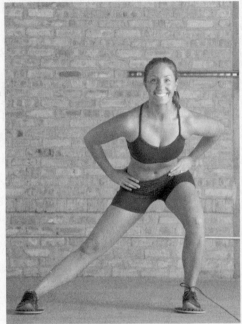

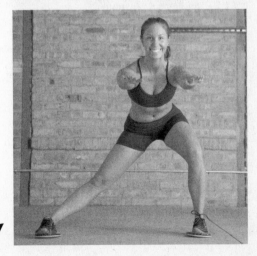

Superadvanced

6. Side Planks with *REVVED*glides

1. Lie on your left elbow on your side with your right foot stacked on top of your left foot.

2. Start out lying on the floor, and then lift up until you are planking on the left side.

3. Place a *REVVED*glide under your right hand.

4. Slowly move your right hand and the *REVVED*glide away from your body, directly in front of your chest, while keeping your hips up.

5. Remember your three count as it applies to this exercise.

6. Pause, then move your hand and the *REVVED*glide as far under the left side of your chest as you can as the hand performs a counterclockwise twist. *Note:* Your body will turn slightly.

7. Breathe comfortably throughout the movement.

8. Do 10 repetitions and repeat on the other side immediately.

Beginner: You may simply hold the side plank until you are ready to add the *REVVED*glide arm movement.

Advanced: Reach your working hand even farther, which will throw you somewhat off balance and require your core to work that much harder.

Superadvanced: Lift your top leg straight up. Keep it there throughout each movement and only lower it when you are done with all 10 repetitions.

This unilateral exercise should take you 1 minute on each side for a total of 2 minutes.

Take 30 seconds for rest and preparation.

Total time: 13 minutes

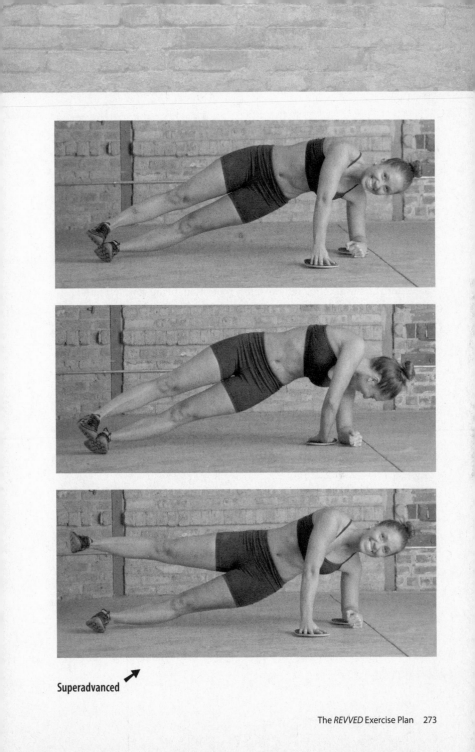

Superadvanced

7. *REVVED*glide Push-Ups

1. Assume the push-up position with the *REVVED*glides under your hands—start on your knees.

2. Make sure that your body is parallel to the floor and that your abdominals are tucked. Imagine you could balance a glass of water on the small of your back even though you are on your knees.

3. Slowly move your left hand about 6 inches to the left and keep it there.

4. Now perform 10 slow push-ups to your three count, with your left arm out and on the *REVVED*glide.

5. After you have completed the tenth repetition, bring your left hand back to the starting position. Then press your right arm out the same distance you did for the left and perform 10 more push-ups.

6. Remember your breathing: Inhale on the way down and exhale on the way up.

_____

Beginner: You may simply perform 20 slow push-ups without the *REVVED*glides. After 10 repetitions, you may rest for about 15 seconds. After you can complete that challenge, then lift up onto your toes for the same number of repetitions.

Advanced: Make the movement more fluid and press your left arm out as you lower to the ground and then slowly bring it back under your shoulder as you press back up to the starting position.

Superadvanced: Press both arms out at the same time as you lower into your push-up, then bring your arms back together as you rise up and squeeze your chest. Rest, then repeat for another set. When you are ready, move up onto your toes. Trust me, it's superadvanced, but you will be shocked when you are both strong *and* lean enough to do it.

_____

This unilateral exercise should take you 1 minute on each side for a total of 2 minutes.

Take 30 seconds for rest and preparation.

Total time: 15½ minutes

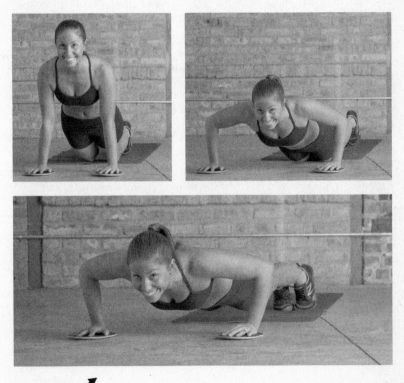

Superadvanced

8. *REVVED*glide Inner-Thigh Squats

1. Stand straight up with your hands on your hips, your feet shoulder-width apart, your toes forward, your knees slightly bent, and your abdominals tucked.

2. Place one *REVVED*glide under each foot.

3. Slowly press both feet out about 2 inches to the side, then bring them back together. Think of your lower body as a pair of scissors that you open up and then clip back together. That's the movement.

4. As you press out, you are performing a partial squat.

5. Inhale on the way out, exhale as you come together.

6. You will be tempted to move quickly, but please abide by your three count because it makes the movement far more effective.

7. Perform 20 repetitions.

———————————

Beginner: You may have to start by simply performing slow squats and progress to the point where you can include the *REVVED*glides. Once you are using the *REVVED*glides, you should first hold on to a chair, counter, or desk for stability.

Advanced: Simply push farther out and slow down the speed to a four, five, or six count.

Superadvanced: As you press out, lower your body until your hamstrings (the backs of your legs) are parallel to the floor. *Note:* You might first attempt this with a chair, counter, or desktop in front of you for stability.

———————————

This exercise should take you 2 minutes.

Take 30 seconds for rest and preparation.

Total time: 18 minutes

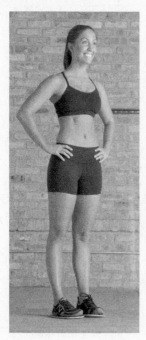

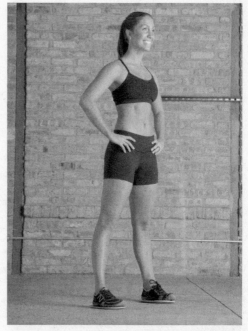

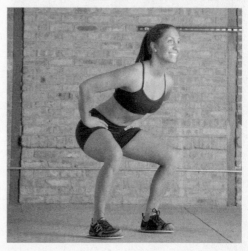

Superadvanced

9. *REVVED*glide Knee-Ins

1. Lie down on the ground in the Pilates plank starting position on your elbows.

2. Place *REVVED*glides under each foot.

3. Start with an inhale, then exhale as you tuck your knees up under your waist.

4. Pause for a moment at the top, then return to the starting position.

5. You will want to rush and not adhere to the "one, one-thousand, two, one-thousand, three, one-thousand" pace. Please don't do that, as this is a very effective core exercise when done slowly.

6. Make sure to keep your chin in alignment at all times. Don't let it tuck too far in, because that is not a favorable position for your neck.

Beginner: You may have to cut down on the range of motion and only move each foot individually by about 6 inches.

Advanced: Slow down to a four, five, or six count. That really intensifies this exercise.

Superadvanced: Come up onto your hands in a push-up position.

This exercise should take you 1 minute.

Take 30 seconds for rest and preparation.

Total time: 19½ minutes

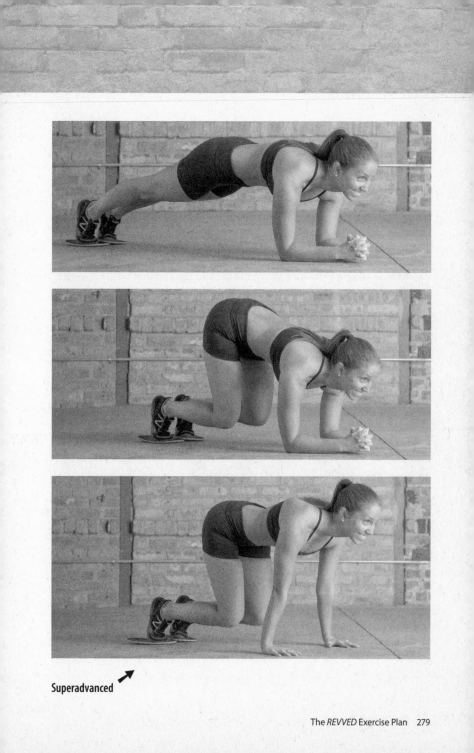

Superadvanced

10. *REVVED* Tricep Push-Ups

1. Start in the push-up plank position, on your knees, with your hands directly under your shoulders.

2. Place *REVVED*glides under each hand.

3. Start inhaling, slide your left arm forward, and drop your right elbow to the ground at a 90-degree angle.

4. Your opposite elbow will bend slightly, giving you increased tension on the stable side and providing tension and overload on both sides.

5. Exhale and pull the *REVVED*glide back to the starting position—use your triceps to really *pull* that arm back in.

6. Keep your entire body stable with your abdominals tucked at all times.

7. Make sure to keep your chin in alignment to create a nice neutral spine.

8. Do 10 repetitions on each side.

Beginner: Perform classic tricep push-ups—10 repetitions, then rest for 30 seconds, and then perform a second set of 10.

Advanced: Perform the original *REVVED* Tricep Push-Up, but start up on your toes with your feet wider than your shoulders.

Superadvanced: Bring your feet closer together, still on your toes, so that your whole body requires more stability throughout the movement.

This unilateral exercise should take you 1 minute on each side for a total of 2 minutes.

Take 30 seconds for rest and preparation.

Total time: 22 minutes

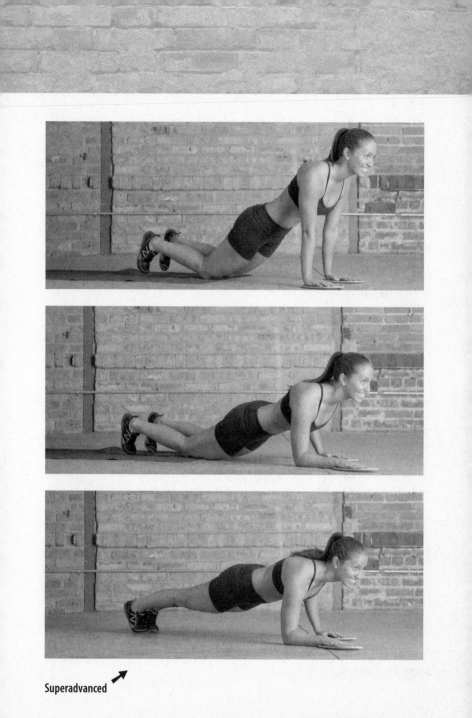

Superadvanced

11. Hamstring Curls with Bridge

1. Lie on your back with your knees up and the *REVVED* glides under each foot.

2. Your hands should be straight up over your head.

3. Lift your glutes up off the floor, then slowly extend your feet until your entire lower body is resting on the floor.

4. As you stay lying on the floor, drag your feet back to the starting position and perform the next repetition.

5. As always, abide by your three count, as that will make the exercise more effective.

6. Begin the exercise with an inhale, then exhale as you lift up and press your feet forward. Then you will inhale as you return to the starting position.

7. Perform 10 repetitions.

Beginner: Simply perform a classic bridge, but stick to the three count.

Advanced: Move slower than a three count and progress to a four, five, or six count, as, once again, time under tension increases intensity.

Superadvanced: Don't let your body lie flat on the floor as you press your feet out. Maintain a position about 1 inch from the floor and then slowly drag your feet back to the starting position.

Superadvanced: As you press your legs out, raise your upper body and arms up as if you are performing a crunch as you execute the bridge.

This exercise should take you 1 minute.

Take 30 seconds for rest and preparation.

Total time: 23½ minutes

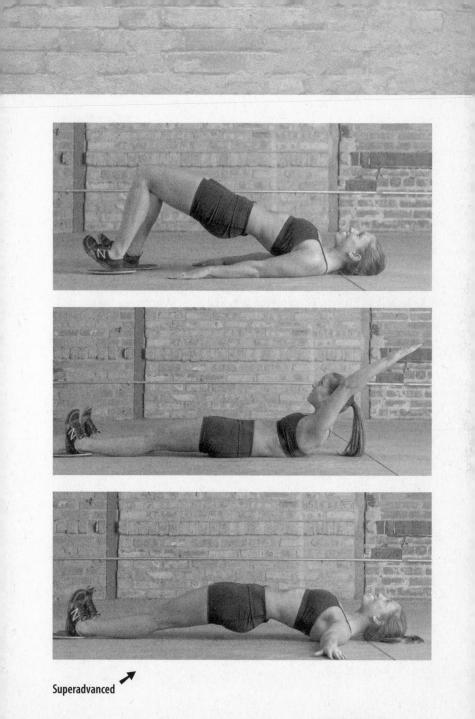

Superadvanced

12. *REVVED* Crunches

1. Start lying on your back with your knees bent and your heels close to your butt with the *REVVED* glides under both heels. Extend your arms over your head parallel with each other.

2. It's very important to tuck your hips and flatten out your lower back so it is pressed firmly and strongly against the floor. This position removes any risk of lower back pain, making room for a stronger core! So first tighten that core, tuck your hips, and create a nice contracted stomach.

3. Then inhale, sliding your feet out so your legs are now straight, with your arms still extended above your head.

4. Exhaling, lift your chest off the floor and bring your hands to your knees, keeping those arms straight and lifting your chest toward the ceiling.

5. Do 10 repetitions.

Beginner: Instead of over your head, place your arms right by your sides or crossed across your chest. This makes less weight for you to pull up.

Advanced: Keep your hands over your head at all times, which will create more tension. Actually squeeze your arms to the sides of your head.

Superadvanced: Slow down to a six count, feel every muscle contracting, and lift higher than ever before with that extra time.

This exercise should take 1 minute.

Take 30 seconds for rest and preparation.

Total time: 25 minutes

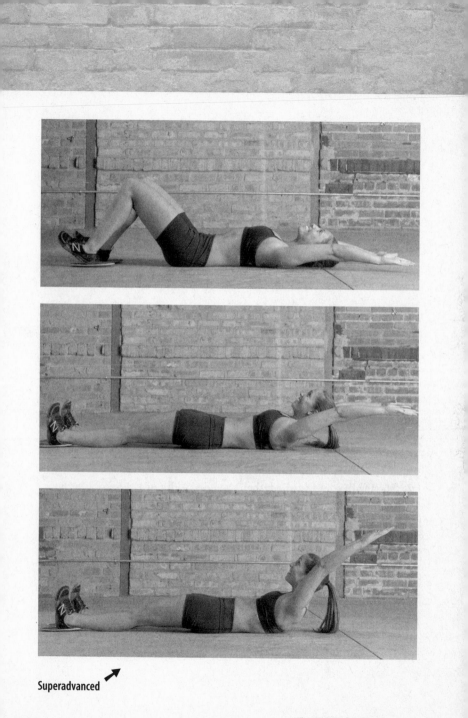

Superadvanced

The following last five exercises are meant to be heart pumping. Now, that's not to say that your heart rate hasn't been elevated, in intervals, throughout this interval-based strength training. The difference is that you will experience an even more rapid heart rate. If at times you are almost out of breath, then you are at the correct intensity. *Note:* The exercises should be performed at the pace of a jumping jack—quick but in very good form.

Each of these exercises should be performed for 1 minute, followed by 30 seconds of rest. If you don't need the full 30 seconds of rest, you haven't worked the HIT exercises hard enough—they are meant to be explosive.

13. **HIT #1: Prone Squats**

1. Assume the Pilates plank position with the *REVVED*glides under each foot.

2. Start with your feet wider than shoulder-width apart, possibly as far out as you can.

3. Quickly pull your feet up close to your shoulders, like a frog getting ready to jump, then go right back to the starting position.

4. Breathe comfortably throughout the movement.

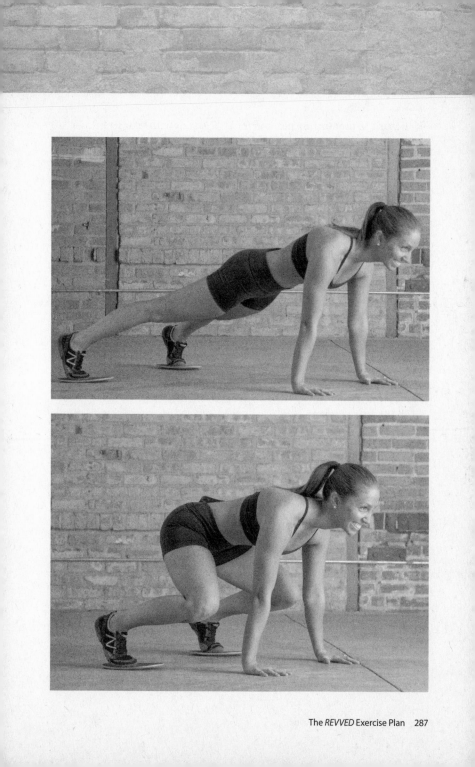

14. HIT #2: Mountain Climbers

1. Return to the starting position for HIT #1, but with your feet closer together.

2. Quickly bring your right foot and knee forward; then as you return to the starting position, bring your left foot and knee forward.

3. This resembles the movement of a mountain climber, which is why it received its name.

4. Don't let your back pitch up. You want to maintain as flat a back as possible to work more of your core.

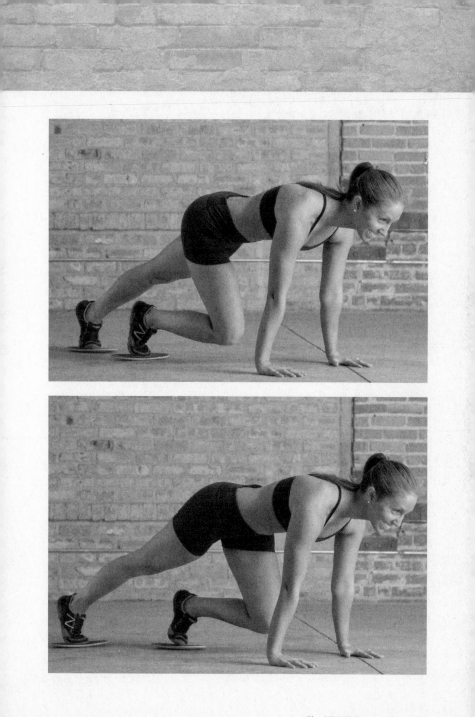

1. Start in the Pilates plank position with *REVVED*glides under both sets of toes.

2. Keep your body completely parallel to the floor at all times.

3. First, press your feet as far apart as possible.

4. Then quickly slide your feet back together and return to the starting position.

5. This movement is fast, but in good form your core and inner thighs should be challenged.

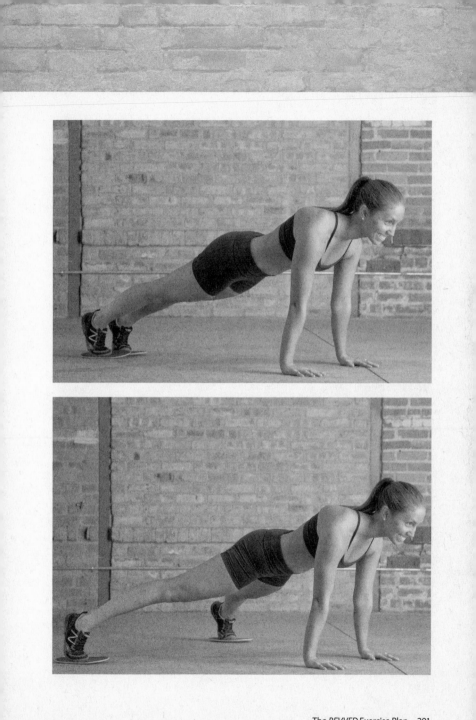

16. HIT #4: Standing Stair Steppers

1. Stand straight up with your knees slightly bent, your feet shoulder-width apart, and your toes forward.

2. Move your right foot forward and your left foot back at the same time.

3. Quickly switch your feet, similar to a rapid cross-country skiing movement.

4. Maintain good posture at all times, and tuck in your abdominals to support your core.

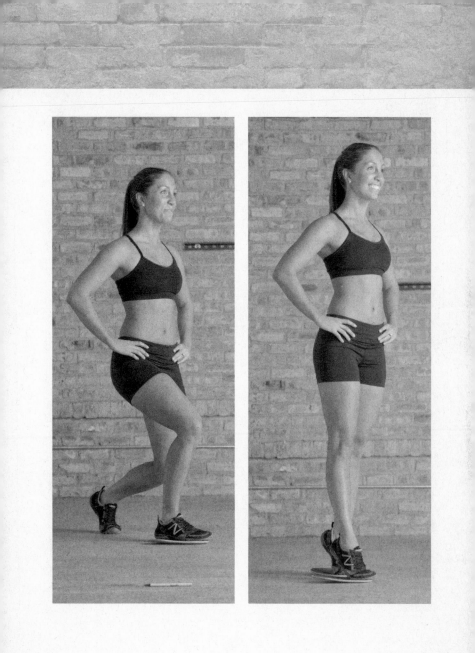

1. Stand straight up with your hands on your hips, your feet shoulder-width apart, your toes forward, your knees slightly bent, and your abdominals tucked.

2. Place one *REVVED*glide under each foot.

3. Quickly press both your feet out about 2 inches, then bring them back together. Think of your lower body as a pair of scissors that you open up and then clip back together.

4. As you press out, you are performing a partial squat.

Note: Yes, this is exactly the same as the advanced movement for the *REVVED* Inner-Thigh Scissors, but you are adding the squat each time and moving much, much faster.

With your final five HIT exercises of 1 minute each, and with 30 seconds of rest between each HIT exercise, you just completed 32 minutes of exercise.

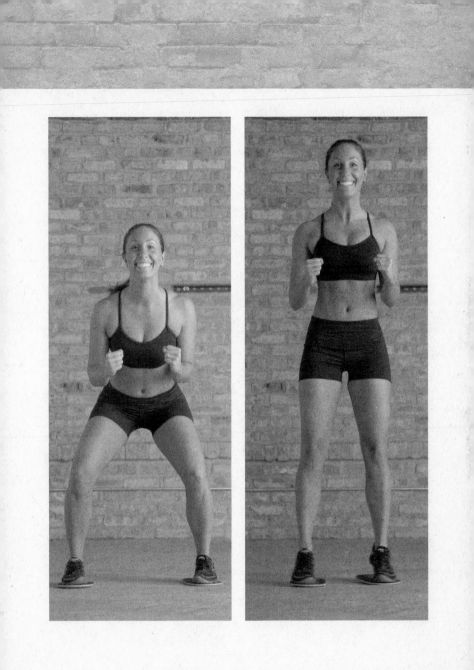

Epilogue

So, we are at the finish line. I hope that you have decided to join the *REV*olution. Maybe it is or maybe it's not the right time for *you*. Timing is a big part of your success on this plan, so don't attempt it when you have a major crisis in the making at work or a difficult period ahead with a child, friend, or other loved one. You know yourself better than anyone else. Choose the time, mark it in ink in your calendar, and off you (and the weight and the fat) will go.

For years I have pitched potential clients at parties, at soccer practice, on the street, you name it. They smile but don't bite. Then, I *finally* get an e-mail, text, or call and the message is simple: "I'm ready." Figure out if you are ready or if you just need some time to let all the information I have given you sink in. Call it your "processing" phase and then decide when you want to take action.

In terms of your processing, please remember the following:

1. Believe in the numbers as they don't lie. If the scale is up, your calories in minus your calories out equal your present body weight. Don't kid yourself. Work your equation.

2. Embrace the Seven *REVVED* Secrets and the role of:

   a. **Muscle.** It *is* the engine of your *REVVED* body.

   b. **Genes.** No, they aren't bad (but odds are your behavior is).

   c. **Sleep.** *So* simple—you snooze, you lose!

   d. **Stress.** No, you probably can't eliminate it, but you can reduce it.

e. **Music.** Allow it to work its magic, and play it often, and sometimes—like first thing in the morning or when you are working out—loud.

f. **Thyroid.** Please get it checked if you believe it may be an issue. Get the data. Data powers reaching your *REVVED* goals.

g. **Human Growth Hormone.** Do everything in your power, like not eating or drinking any liquid calories two hours before bed, to enhance it.

3. Never, ever cleanse again. *Only* cleanse if your goal is weight gain and a reduction in your *REVVED* results. Don't fall into this oh-so-popular trend that can leave you doomed to gain weight, diminish your metabolism, and make permanent weight and fat loss all but impossible. . . . until you go on this plan.

4. Live by *The Ultimate Diet* REVolution eating rules and:

a. Reverse your caloric intake and eat the majority of your calories before 3:00 PM and start with a big breakfast.

b. Eat on a schedule as your body, mind, and hormones *love* schedules.

c. Stop the snacking and only allow it after interval-based strength-training. Don't even call it a snack. Call it a recovery meal.

d. Stop shunning fat as it is your BFF when it comes to weight loss and satiety. Just make it the right fat combined with your meals.

e. Spice it up as spices are packed with antioxidants, tip satiety, and make food taste *good*.

5. Shun liquid calories, even those from alcohol, for these first 28 days. Then, reintroduce alcohol when you are ready but only in a portion-controlled manner. Power up on tea as it, well, powers *REVVED* results.

6. Believe me when I say that the only style of exercise you ever want to perform is interval-based strength-training. At the end of it, accelerate your *REVVED* metabolism with the HIT training routine

I taught you. You will literally watch the fat melt away as you uncover long, lean sexy muscles you probably thought you would never see.

I've said throughout this book that I have decades of experience when it comes to weight loss, specifically fat loss, and more important, *permanent* weight loss. That's my goal for you. This isn't a gimmick or a "quick fix" as we have determined that these don't work.

Let me take you back to that somewhat unpleasant statistic from the first page of the introduction: The success rate at weight loss is an incredibly low 5 percent. If you have this book in your hands, odds are you are sitting with the rest of the 95 percent wondering, "What's wrong with me? Why can't I lose the weight and then keep it off?"

The reason is simple: You tried the wrong eating plan, almost positively the wrong exercise plan, and you did it in an environment of imbalances—hormones, sleep deprivation, and raging stress. Don't blame yourself. Blame the lack of knowledge, or better yet, blame the media, the "false" claims, and the big business that comes with American's deep desire to lose weight.

I urge you, join my *REVol*ution. Join Diane Sawyer, Hugh Jackman, and the hundreds, no thousands, maybe hundreds of thousands, that I have helped lose weight and achieve incredible shape.

It's here. It's your choice. It's only 28 days away.

It's *The Ultimate Diet* REV*olution. . . .*

Acknowledgments

I would like to start by thanking my team at Harper One, Nancy Hancock, my editor, and Suzanne Wickham, my publicist. We hit the *New York Times* bestseller list with our first book together, *The Petite Advantage Diet,* and then had a good run. I certainly hope we do the same with this book. Okay, I'm going to be honest and replace the "I certainly hope" with "I know we will." Thanks for all your hard work and support.

Then I would like to thank my team at Jim Karas Personal Training under the leadership of Phil Chung and Justin Bomkamp. Together we have identified, refined, and practiced many of the techniques in this book. We stand, as a team, committed to enabling our Chicago and New York clients to achieve results far beyond their expectations. Just know how much I appreciate your passion, professionalism, and dedication to excellence.

I must again thank Juliette Britton who beautifully crafted our *REVVED* Eating Plan according to my specifications. Not only did you help me create a success-driven weight loss eating plan, but your creativity and research-driven recommendations even inspired me to think about—and then make—smarter choices for me *and* for my family.

Speaking of my family, I must always thank my two children, Olivia and Evan. Olivia, you continue to inspire me with your passion and dedication to gymnastics. Given that you are the junior Olympic champion (that is a moment I will never forget when your name popped up on the top of the leader board) and headed to the University of Michigan to compete for them in the fall of 2015, I'm happy to say that passion and dedication are paying off. Please know that's not always the case, but I truly hope you continue to "lead with your heart," love the sport that has given you such joy, and find the right balance in life. I know you can do it.

Evan, whom I call "Baba," is like my shaman. He gives me important "life" advice (which I don't solicit but appear to frequently need), and he just turned fourteen. If I'd had his wisdom at that age . . . Evan, you're smart, driven (like your sister and father), funny, creative, and a fiercely competitive athlete. I don't really know where you are headed in life as you are just finishing eighth grade, but I'm sure it will never be dull. Look, you made me go on the fastest roller coaster in the world in Abu Dhabi (and after that, I'm done as I went out with the best). That might be an indication of your future to come.

A special thank-you to a few important members of my "extended" family: Jana DeLancey, Lisa Huston, Regina Walker, and Vijay Vasista. All four of you have supported me not only through this book project but through many of my life's frequent ups and downs (will it ever calm down?). Thank you for listening, thank you for caring, and thank you for the sometimes-needed bottomless glass of white wine.

Finally, JNA, I think you know . . .

Notes

Introduction

1. http://www.cdc.gov/nchs/fastats/overwt.htm.
2. http://aje.oxfordjournals.org/content/158/1/85.full; and http://nymag.com/restaurants/features/breakfast/47396/index1.html.
3. http://health.yahoo.net/experts/dayinhealth/surprising-dangers-skipping-breakfast.
4. http://health.yahoo.net/experts/dayinhealth/surprising-dangers-skipping-breakfast.
5. http://ajcn.nutrition.org/content/82/1/222S.full.

Chapter 1: *REVVED* by the Numbers

1. Collins English Dictionary; and http://www.thefreedictionary.com/metabolism.
2. Collins English Dictionary; and http://www.thefreedictionary.com/basal+metabolism.
3. http://www.nmh.org/nm/metabolic-testing.
4. http://abcnews.go.com/GMA/Weekend/exercise-calorie-counters-work/story?id=9966500.

Chapter 2: The Seven Secrets of *REVVED*

1. http://articles.latimes.com/2011/may/16/health/la-he-fitness-muscle-myth-20110516.
2. http://www.nytimes.com/2013/07/19/health/overweight-maybe-you-really-can-blame-your-metabolism.html?pagewanted=all&_r=1&
3. Claude Bouchard et al., "The Response to Long-Term Overfeeding in Identical Twins," *New England Journal of Medicine* 322 (May 1990): 1477–82.
4. http://articles.mercola.com/sites/articles/archive/2012/02/13/scientists-find-brown-fat-to-help-lose-weight.aspx.
5. http://www.webmd.com/diet/features/the-truth-about-fat.
6. http://healthland.time.com/2011/11/02/gym-vs-genes-how-exercise-trumps-obesity-genes/#ixzz2eG34yZY0.
7. http://healthland.time.com/2011/11/02/gym-vs-genes-how-exercise-trumps-obesity-genes/#ixzz2eG34yZY0.
8. http://diabetes.diabetesjournals.org/content/early/2008/07/03/db08-0214.full.pdf
9. http://www.npr.org/blogs/health/2010/04/exercise_trumps_gene_in_teen_o.html.

10. http://www.npr.org/blogs/health/2010/04/exercise_trumps_gene_in_teen_o.html.

11. http://www.ncbi.nlm.nih.gov/pmc/articles/PMC1991337/.

12. http://biology.about.com/od/anatomy/p/pituitary-gland.htm.

13. http://www.precisionnutrition.com/sleep-prevents-ffm-loss.

14. http://www.news-medical.net/health/What-is-Leptin.aspx.

15. http://www.ncbi.nlm.nih.gov/pmc/articles/PMC535701/.

16. http://wellnessmama.com/5356/cravings-fix-your-leptin.

17. http://www.ncbi.nlm.nih.gov/pubmed/15583226

18. National Sleep Foundation, "Hungry for Sleep," *Fitness Matters* 11, no. 5 (September–October 2005): 11.

19. National Sleep Foundation, "Hungry for Sleep," 11.

20. http://www.mayoclinic.com/health/insomnia/DS00187/DSECTION = coping-and-support.

21. http://www.huffingtonpost.com/2013/05/17/alcohol-side-effects-drinking-sleep_n_3286434.html.

22. http://articles.mercola.com/sites/articles/archive/2012/02/13/scientists-find-brown-fat-to-help-lose-weight.aspx.

23. David Dinges, chief of the Division of Sleep and Chronobiology at the University of Pennsylvania School of Medicine.

24. http://health.usnews.com/health-news/managing-your-healthcare/sleep/articles/2010/08/04/sleep-deprived-heres-how-to-recover.

25. "A Field Guide to the Perfect Nap," *Wall Street Journal*, Personal Journal, September 3, 2013, sec. D1, p. 1.

26. http://www.precisionnutrition.com/sleep-prevents-ffm-loss.

27. http://www.mayoclinic.com/health/stress/SR00001.

28. "How Much Stress Does It Take to Make a Man Go Grey," *Best Life* (October 2008): 20.

29. David Schipper, "Outsmart Your Stomach," *Men's Health* (October 2008): 137.

30. Thea Singer, "Calming the Fat Away," *O, The Oprah Magazine* (May 1, 2012): 148.

31. http://www.paulwesselmann.com/

32. http://musiced.org.uk/teachers/powerofmusic/pom3.html.

33. http://news.menshealth.com/how-itunes-can-cure-depression/.

34. Baltimore Hospital, "Healing Aspects of Music Physically and Medicinally," http://cc.ysu.edu/-s0133456/healing_aspects_of_music_physically.htm.

35. Robert E. Krout, "Music Listening to Facilitate Relaxation and Promote Wellness," *Arts in Psychotherapy* 34, no. 2 (2007): 134–141.

36. http://www.bbc.co.uk/wales/raiseyourgame/sites/motivation/psychedup/pages/costas_karageorghis.shtml

37. http://www.thatsfit.com/2008/05/13/strong-songs-score-strength-training-success.

38. http://my.clevelandclinic.org/disorders/hyperthyroidism/hic_thyroid_disease.aspx.

39. http://www.foxnews.com/health/2013/08/29/1-signs-your-thyroid-isnt-working-right/.

40. http://www.telegraph.co.uk/health/healthnews/7940957/Women-suffer-headaches-more-than-men.html.

41. http://www.thebodywellusa.com/blog/dr-mike-carraghers-top-10-ways-to-increase-your-human-growth-hormone-hgh-levels-naturally/.

42. http://livingsuperhuman.com/6-ways-to-boost-hgh-levels-naturally/#sthash.gm9AMRTz.dpuf.

Chapter 3: The *REV*elation

1. http://www.gallup.com/poll/157505/americans-exercising-slightly-2012.aspx

2. http://fisher.osu.edu/~schroeder_9/AMIS900/Manski1993.pdf.

Chapter 4: The *REVVED* Eating Rules

1. http://www.weightlossresources.co.uk/calories/calorie_needs/secret-eaters.htm.
2. http://ajcn.nutrition.org/content/83/2/211.full.
3. http://thechart.blogs.cnn.com/2013/01/29/meal-times-may-affect-weight-loss-success/.
4. http://www.ncbi.nlm.nih.gov/pubmed/19730426.
5. http://www.webmd.com/diet/features/lose-weight-eat-breakfast.
6. http://www.webmd.com/diet/features/lose-weight-eat-breakfast.
7. http://www.dailymail.co.uk/health/article-2202590/Eating-high-fat-diet-prevent-obesity-improve-metabolism.html.
8. http://www.dailymail.co.uk/health/article-2202590/Eating-high-fat-diet-prevent-obesity-improve-metabolism.html.
9. http://diabetes.niddk.nih.gov/dm/pubs/insulinresistance/#what.
10. http://drmikehart.ca/2013/07/30/the-other-side-of-saturated-fats-health-benefits-of-a-fat-rich-diet/
11. http://www.naturalnews.com/026808_oil_coconut.html.
12. http://www.naturalnews.com/026808_oil_coconut.html#ixzz2dBHIqDLr.
13. http://www.hailmerry.com/blog/2012/02/difference-between-short-chains-long-chain-fats/.
14. http://www.ncbi.nlm.nih.gov/pubmed/18602429.
15. http://www.webmd.com/diet/features/increase-your-metabolism-start-losing-fat?page=3.
16. http://www.ifosprogram.com/Consumer-Reports.aspx; and http://www.webmd.cFish om/diet/features/increase-your-metabolism-start-losing-fat?page=3.
17. http://www.ncbi.nlm.nih.gov/pubmed/10375057.
18. http://www.ncbi.nlm.nih.gov/pubmed/18469287; and http://workoutsolutions.blogspot.com/2011/07/improved-appetite-control-and-satiety.html.
19. http://ajcn.nutrition.org/content/83/2/211.abstract.
20. http://www.eurekalert.org/pub_releases/2010-04/epr-eef040210.php.
21. http://www.rejuvenation-science.com/n_pinolenic-acid_satiety.html
22. http://www.fitnessmagazine.com/recipes/healthy-eating/superfoods/fat-fighting-superfoods/?page=3.
23. http://www.fitnessmagazine.com/recipes/healthy-eating/superfoods/fat-fighting-superfoods/?page=6.
24. http://healthyeating.sfgate.com/vitamins-burn-fat-increase-metabolism-5876.html.
25. http://healthhubs.net/weight-loss/vitamin-c-associated-with-lower-bmi-body-fat-levels/.
26. http://www.ncbi.nlm.nih.gov/pubmed/15930480.
27. http://www.healthaliciousness.com/articles/vitamin-C.php; and http://www.fitnessmagazine.com/recipes/healthy-eating/superfoods/fat-fighting-superfoods/?page=5.

Chapter 5: Liquid *REVVED*

1. http://www.amypaturel.com/articles/article_pdf_155.pdf.
2. http://www.amypaturel.com/articles/article_pdf_155.pdf.
3. http://www.webmd.com/diet/features/water-stress-reduction?page=1
4. http://www.ncbi.nlm.nih.gov/pubmed/20336685.
5. http://www.lifehack.org/articles/lifestyle/11-benefits-lemon-water-you-didnt-know-about.html.
6. http://www.webmd.com/fitness-exercise/features/water-for-exercise-fitness.
7. Read more at http://www.voxxi.com/water-rich-foods/#ixzz2cM8raEKm; and http://www.voxxi.com/water-rich-foods/.

8. http://www.fitday.com/fitness-articles/nutrition/healthy-eating/uncovering-the-truth-can-drinking-green-tea-help-with-weight-loss.html#b.

9. http://www.webmd.com/food-recipes/news/20040525/white-tea-beats-green-tea-at-killing-germs.

10. http://www.huffingtonpost.com/2012/07/25/half-of-americans-drink-soda-everyday-consumption_n_1699540.html.

11. http://www.huffingtonpost.com/2012/07/25/half-of-americans-drink-soda-everyday-consumption_n_1699540.html.

12. Tucker-Falconer, R. and Mattes, R.D. (2013) "Satiation, satiety: the puzzle of solids and liquids." In: *Satiation, satiety and the control of food intake.* Blundell, J. and Bellisle, F. Ed(s). Woodhead Pub Ltd., Cambridge, UK.

13. http://herbalwater.typepad.com/ayalas_herbal_water/2012/01/study-shows-liquid-calories-trick-body-and-mind-to-overeat.html.

14. http://herbalwater.typepad.com/ayalas_herbal_water/2012/01/study-shows-liquid-calories-trick-body-and-mind-to-overeat.html.

15. http://www.washingtonpost.com/wp-dyn/articles/A30903-2004Dec28.html.

16. http://www.washingtonpost.com/wp-dyn/articles/A30903-2004Dec28.html.

17. http://www.prevention.com/weight-loss/weight-loss-tips/10-diet-and-fitness-rumors-slow-weight-loss.

18. http://articles.mercola.com/sites/articles/archive/2012/02/20/can-diet-soda-increase-stroke-risk.aspx.

19. http://in.reuters.com/article/2008/02/11/idINIndia-31866220080211.

Chapter 6: The *REVVED* Eating Plan

1. http://naldc.nal.usda.gov/download/33230/PDF.

2. http://news.psu.edu/story/140750/2003/05/01/research/pasture-ized-poultry.

3. http://www.webmd.com/cholesterol-management/news/20080111/heartier-benefits-seen-from-oatmeal.

4. http://www.ncbi.nlm.nih.gov/pubmed/17490954.

5. http://www.health.harvard.edu/fhg/updates/Microwave-cooking-and-nutrition.shtml.

6. http://www.foodnavigator.com/Science-Nutrition/Oregano-rosemary-extracts-promise-omega-3-preservation.

7. http://www.nutraingredients-usa.com/Research/Antioxidant-rich-cocoa-shows-short-term-heart-benefits-Harvard-review.

8. http://www.ncbi.nlm.nih.gov/pubmed/16500874.

9. http://www.huffingtonpost.com/paul-spector-md/sugar-substitutes_b_1515004.html; and http://www.ncbi.nlm.nih.gov/pubmed/18298259.

10. http://naldc.nal.usda.gov/download/33230/PDF.

11. http://news.psu.edu/story/140750/2003/05/01/research/pasture-ized-poultry.

12. http://www.webmd.com/cholesterol-management/news/20080111/heartier-benefits-seen-from-oatmeal.

13. http://www.ncbi.nlm.nih.gov/pubmed/17490954.

14. http://www.health.harvard.edu/fhg/updates/Microwave-cooking-and-nutrition.shtml.

15. http://www.foodnavigator.com/Science-Nutrition/Oregano-rosemary-extracts-promise-omega-3-preservation.

16. http://www.ncbi.nlm.nih.gov/pubmed/16500874.

17. http://www.huffingtonpost.com/paul-spector-md/sugar-substitutes_b_1515004.html; and http://www.ncbi.nlm.nih.gov/pubmed/18298259.

Chapter 7: The *REVVED* Exercise Rules

1. http://www.menshealth.com/fitness/spartacus-workout-science.
2. http://www.ncbi.nlm.nih.gov/pubmed/18616997.
3. http://well.blogs.nytimes.com/2009/10/14/phys-ed-does-exercise-boost-immunity/.
4. http://www.menshealth.com/health/effects-air-pollution.
5. http://www.menshealth.com/fitness/spartacus-workout-science
6. http://link.springer.com/article/10.1007 percent2Fs00421–001–0568-y.
7. http://www.harpersbazaar.com/beauty/health-wellness-articles/is-spinning-making-you-fat-0913.

Index

About the Author

Jim Karas is a lifestyle expert who combines a degree from the Wharton School of Business with more than twenty years of unparalleled success in helping people look and feel their very best.

Jim is the author of the #1 *New York Times* bestseller *The Business Plan for the Body*, the *New York Times* bestsellers, *The Cardio-Free Diet, The 7-Day Energy Surge*, and *The Petite Advantage Diet*, as well as *Flip The Switch*.

Jim has been an *ABC News* contributor (he helped Diane Sawyer lose more than 25 pounds) and the fitness expert on *Good Morning America*. He is frequently seen on *The Dr. Oz Show* and *The View*, and for three years he hosted "Couch Potatoes" on *ABC News Now*. Jim has served as a contributing editor for *Good Housekeeping* magazine and has written feature articles for countless other national publications, including "O" *The Oprah Magazine*.

Jim is a widely sought after as a keynote speaker for many of the country's most prominent corporations and organizations such as Oprah's O You!; Blue Cross, Blue Shield; the Chicago Board of Trade; Fortune Brands; Kraft Foods; Wrigley and Young; and World Presidents' Organization, to name a few.

Since 1987, he continues to run Jim Karas Personal Training in both Chicago and New York. *Allure* magazine named him "One of the Best Personal Trainers in the Country."

Jim sits on the advisory board of Performance Trust Capital Partners and is the chairman of the Philanthropic Advisory Council for the Osher Center for Integrative Medicine at Northwestern University.